yoga

beats the blues

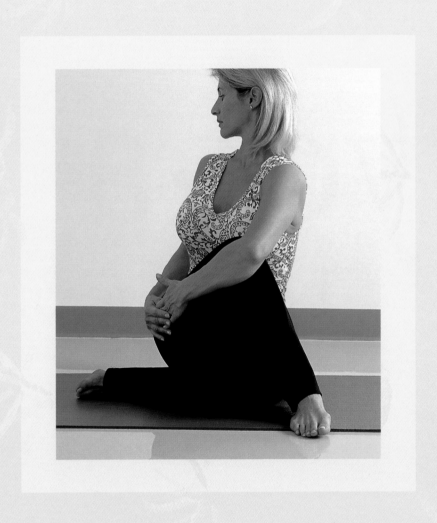

yoga
beats the blues

Boost Your Mood, Energy, and Concentration

with Easy 5-Minute, 10-Minute, and 20-Minute Yoga Routines

Donna Raskin

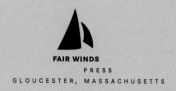

FAIR WINDS
PRESS
GLOUCESTER, MASSACHUSETTS

First published in the USA in 2003 by
Fair Winds Press
33 Commercial Street
Gloucester, MA 01930

Library of Congress Cataloging-in-Publication Data available

ISBN 1-59233-022-3

10 9 8 7 6 5 4 3 2 1

Book design by Yee Design
Photography by Bobbie Bush Photography, www.bobbiebush.com

Printed and bound in China

*The information in this book is for educational purposes only. It is not intended
to replace the advice of a physician or medical practitioner. Please see your health care
provider before beginning any new health program.*

For Pat Brown

contents

introduction

My Story

As much as we try to avoid them, the blues are a natural part of life. I've had everything from the "I-need-to-lose-10-pounds-in-two-days" blues to "What-is-the-reason-for-my-existence?" middle of the night despair. I've even experienced an overwhelming pile of life stresses that most people only fear will fall on them.

Here's what happened: Between June 2000 and August 2001, I had a baby, moved across the country, was left by my son's father, lost my job, and then moved back across the country with the baby when I got a new job. A baby, two jobs, two major moves, and a breakup. Fourteen months and six major life changes, one on top of the other.

Sometimes, when I tell people about that time in my life, they look at me like I'm a walking miracle because I not only survived what experts say are some of the most stressful events that happen in our lifetime, but I actually felt, for the most part, fairly secure and hopeful.

"You should be lying on the couch with a bottle of vodka," one of my friends said to me that year. "You would have every right to do that."

But I never once did that. I had—and continue to have—a secret ally that not only minimized the stress I felt, but also helped me thrive both physically and emotionally.

What keeps me sane, happy, and calm is yoga. I have practiced yoga for 25 years, ever since I found a copy of Indra Devi's book *Yoga for Americans* in my grandmother's attic when I was a teenager. Featuring a forward by Gloria Swanson, the silent screen star who went on to portray Norma Desmond in the classic film *Sunset Boulevard, Yoga for Americans*—like the book you're holding—was a compilation of poses and instructions designed to help people learn this 2,000-year-old practice that includes poses, breathing, and meditation.

Even back then, when I struggled to balance on one foot and push myself into a tangle of bent knees and crossed arms—and when I didn't know anyone else who practiced—yoga made me happy. But more than that, over the years yoga has taught me how to bring that same happiness to any situation—even the toughest ones, such as break-ups and job loss. When I look back over the past 25 years, I realize that yoga has given me easy-to-master physical and emotional tools that help me maintain a sense of serenity. It can do the same for you.

It's not that I don't get the blues. I do. I feel scared, worried, and anxious. I even know that things will happen in the future that will bring those feelings back to me when I least expect it. But throughout all of my fears and worries, yoga has helped me focus on the serenity that always resides in me, no matter what is going on around me—be it chaos in world events or my own feelings taking me for a ride.

It's possible that you're reading this and thinking that your blues are more acute than mine were. But about eight years ago I did suffer from a debilitating case of anxiety and depression—the kind that put me in the hospital and on medication for a few months—so I can assure you that I've felt the full range of blues. If you're wondering where yoga was back then, when I needed it most, I will tell you that my depression at that point was so far gone that yoga alone was not enough to help me. I explain more about other solutions that are needed in very serious cases of depression and anxiety on page 20.

My yoga practice—a combination of breathwork, poses, and meditation—has helped me create a program that not only helps me feel better when I am sad or scared, but also helps me stave off future bouts of sadness.

Yoga has not been studied by the medical profession as thoroughly as other health protocols have been, but it has been scientifically proven to relieve the symptoms of both depression and anxiety. Jon Kabat-Zinn, Dean Ornish, and other researchers and physicians have found that yoga, as well as meditation, improve health and decrease the symptoms of anxiety and depression. A study conducted by Eric Hoffman, Ph.D., in Scandinavia, measured brain wave activity in Kriya yoga students. The research showed that, scientifically speaking, the brains of the yoga students were more relaxed after a yoga class than before it. Yoga students will often tell you they feel more relaxed after class (and that they then carry that relaxation into the rest of their lives) and more research is beginning to independently support those observations.

I can personally attest to yoga's powers of healing and relaxation. Whether you're feeling blue due to a serious change in your life or simply because you're overwhelmed by your responsibilities, yoga can help you feel more centered and strong.

Yoga doesn't ask you to contort your body into weird poses, nor does it force you to adopt a new religion or start chanting. Instead, a true yoga practice only asks you to let go of the unpleasant and ineffective ways that you are speaking to yourself and moving your body. It asks you to learn how to bring your body together with your highest spiritual self. Once you can do this—once you can let go of your judgment and enjoy yourself, whether you're in a difficult pose or an easy, relaxing pose—there is a good chance that you will be able to find peace of mind no matter what situation you are in. And that peace of mind is the key to happiness.

You Are Not Your Blues

The way I see it, "the blues" or, in more clinical terms, depression and anxiety, are the opposite of happiness. Happiness is a feeling that any of us can experience, even though we each describe it a little differently. For me, happiness feels like a little river in which everything is flowing smoothly; things neither move too rapidly nor too calmly. I'm happy when I'm not obsessing on a specific thought such as "I have to lose 5 pounds" or "How am I going to pay that bill?" and I'm also not overwhelmed with sad or negative feelings.

On the flip side, when I'm happy, I'm also not frantic with energy. As much as I enjoy the adrenaline rush I get from teaching yoga, let's say, or performing music (I like to sing), those situations give me a little bit of stress, too. It's nerve-wracking to be in front of an audience when I perform, and when I'm teaching I have a lot to remember while I simultaneously have to pay attention to a lot of people. So even though I enjoy teaching, I can't say it always makes me happy.

At the same time, even when I'm happy inside—when the words are flowing smoothly and no negative thoughts are intruding on my delicate brain—the world sometimes asks me to pay attention to upsetting things: violence against children, illness, people who suffer from addictions. Happiness is not about what is outside of you. If you have to depend on the world's cooperation, I can tell you right now, you won't ever feel happy.

But little can be accomplished—even against the harshness of the world—without happiness. This is because part of happiness (a key part, in fact) is feeling hopeful. You must believe, somewhere inside you, that good will prevail, that joy will find you, and that something fabulous is just around the corner, especially if it doesn't happen to be sitting in your lap or residing in your soul right at this very moment.

Why am I waxing philosophical about happiness and pain, negativity and hope? Because it is of the utmost importance for you to understand that *you are not your blues.*

Life hands us both lots to be sad and scared about and lots to be joyful about. The healthiest among us appreciate each experience for what it is and feel each feeling that comes up without letting those feelings overtake each part of our lives. When we are healthy, our feelings are a part of our whole selves, rather than our lives being held hostage by our feelings.

We know depression and anxiety are present when we are doing things that we enjoy, such as walking, dancing, lying on a beach, riding a motorcycle, or doing any of the millions of things there are for us to do in this lifetime, but we still don't feel happy. In fact, if you check out "Symptoms of Clinical Depression" on page 14, you'll see that not being able to enjoy activities that previously made you happy is one sign that something is wrong.

1. Persistent sad, anxious, or "empty" mood

2. Sleeping too much or too little; middle of the night or early morning waking

3. Reduced appetite and weight loss, or increased appetite and weight gain

4. Loss of pleasure and interest in activities once enjoyed, including sex

5. Restlessness and irritability

6. Persistent physical symptoms that do not respond to treatment (such as chronic pain or digestive disorders)

7. Difficulty concentrating, remembering, or making decisions

8. Fatigue or loss of energy

9. Feeling guilty, hopeless, or worthless

10. Thoughts of suicide or death

If you have five or more of these symptoms for two weeks or more, you could have clinical depression and should see your doctor or a qualified mental health professional for help.

Clinical depression, which includes a major depressive disorder, manic depression and dysthymia (a milder, longer-lasting form of depression), affects more than 19 million Americans each year, according to the National Institutes of Health. Depression can occur in anyone, at any age, and to people of any race or ethnic group. Still, despite its prevalence, depression is never a "normal" part of life, no matter what your age, gender, or health situation.

Similarly, anxiety disorders develop from a complex set of risk factors, including genetics, brain chemistry, personality, and life events. And let's face it, there's a lot in this world that makes us nervous for a good reason. Whether it's job insecurity or violence in society, it's easy to find reasons to be nervous.

And yet, just because there are reasons to be nervous doesn't mean that you have to be. Of course, healthy nervousness—when we realize we need to protect ourselves in proportion to the danger we're in—is beneficial.

However, when we're safe and we still feel scared and anxious, or if anxiety keeps us from taking risks or moving forward with our lives, then we need to deal with the anxiety as an illness that isn't based on realistic fears.

Anxiety disorders are highly treatable, yet only about one-third of those suffering from them receive treatment. Too many people resist treatment because they believe that depression and anxiety aren't serious, that they can treat the disorders themselves, or worse, that these are personal weaknesses rather than serious medical illnesses. But none of these things are true. Depression and anxiety are natural responses to stress, and they can also be illnesses that are easily treated and cured.

In other words, you don't have to live with the blues.

How Come I Feel So Blue?

Sometimes we know exactly why we feel down: Someone has broken our heart, we can't find a job that pays enough or makes us feel worthwhile, or we're overwhelmed by a number of little things that cause us to feel helpless. Other times, depression seems to come out of nowhere. Things are fine, but we aren't.

According to the National Institute of Mental Health, a number of factors can create a depressed mood.

BIOLOGY. People with depression typically have too little or too much of certain brain chemicals called "neurotransmitters." Changes in these brain chemicals may cause or contribute to clinical depression.

COGNITION. People with negative thinking patterns and low self-esteem are more likely to develop clinical depression.

GENDER. Women experience clinical depression at nearly twice the rate that men do. While the reasons for this are still unclear, they may include the hormonal changes women go through during menstruation, pregnancy, childbirth, and menopause, as well as the stress caused by the multiple responsibilities that women have.

ILLNESS AND MEDICATION. Clinical depression is more likely to occur in conjunction with certain illnesses, such as heart disease, cancer, Parkinson's, diabetes, Alzheimer's, and hormonal disorders. Some medications can also bring on depression as an unwanted side effect.

GENETICS. A family history of clinical depression increases the risk of developing the illness.

SPECIFIC SITUATIONS. Difficult life events, including divorce, financial problems, or the death of a loved one, can contribute to clinical depression.

Likewise, anxiety takes on many forms (see "Types of Anxiety Disorders" on page 17), but each form can also be caused by one or more of the situations listed above.

TYPES OF ANXIETY DISORDERS
from the National Institute of Mental Health

GENERALIZED ANXIETY DISORDER. Excessive, unrealistic worry that lasts six months or more. When an adult has this, she may worry about her health, money, or career. Other symptoms include trembling, muscular aches, insomnia, abdominal upsets, dizziness, and irritability.

OBSESSIVE-COMPULSIVE DISORDER (OCD). When persistent, recurring thoughts or obsessions plague someone, they are suffering from OCD. Their worries are caused by exaggerated anxiety or fears. Some common obsessions include being contaminated by germs, fears of behaving improperly, or acting violently. The obsessive thoughts often lead sufferers to perform rituals or routines, such as washing hands, repeating phrases, or hoarding to relieve their anxiety. They perform these rituals compulsively, hence the name of the disorder.

PANIC DISORDER. Severe panic attacks feel like real, physical symptoms to the sufferer. A person may feel like he or she is having a heart attack or going crazy. They may feel heart palpitations, chest pain or discomfort, sweating, trembling, tingling sensations, a feeling of choking, fear of dying, fear of losing control, or feelings of unreality. People who suffer from panic attacks often develop agoraphobia (fear of being outside of a familiar place) because they are afraid they will have a panic attack in front of other people.

POST-TRAUMATIC STRESS DISORDER (PTSD). Although most commonly associated with war veterans, anyone can suffer from PTSD. It usually occurs after someone has survived a traumatic event, such as a sexual or physical assault, witnessing a death, the unexpected death of a loved one, or a natural disaster. The main symptoms are consistent memories of the event (such as flashbacks and nightmares), avoidance behaviors (such as avoiding places related to the trauma), emotional numbing (detachment from others), difficulty sleeping, irritability, and poor concentration.

SOCIAL PHOBIA OR SOCIAL ANXIETY DISORDER (SAD). SAD is characterized by extreme anxiety over being judged by others or behaving in a way that might cause embarrassment or ridicule. This intense anxiety may lead to avoidance behavior. Physical symptoms associated with this disorder include heart palpitations, faintness, blushing, and profuse sweating.

SPECIFIC PHOBIAS. A person with a specific phobia suffers from an intense fear reaction to a specific object or situation (such as spiders, dogs, or heights). The level of fear is usually inappropriate to the situation and is recognized by the sufferer as being irrational. This inordinate fear can lead to the avoidance of common, everyday situations.

How and Why Yoga Helps Depression and Anxiety

"The solution is spiritual and it has nothing to do with the problem."

—Anne Lamott

In my experience, one of the most dangerous misconceptions about depression is that people suffering with this illness can "think themselves out of it." Depressed people struggle with their efforts to think through their feelings, while their friends and family often encourage them to just "get over it" and think differently.

It is almost impossible to think differently when your mood can't reach a place that is happy or positive. Moods and thoughts are inextricably linked. When you feel good, it's easy to interpret your experiences and history as positive. But when you feel sad and especially hopeless, any experience can be construed as negative.

It's easy to forget that you were once a happy person—or that you have the ability to be a happy person—when you feel depressed. Your thinking contributes in a large part to how you feel, and part of the disease is an inability to think clearly about life and yourself. This inability leads to feeling very sad.

It's a bad spiral. You think bad thoughts that make you feel bad, which then makes you so physically incapacitated with the symptoms of depression that you cannot lift yourself out of the spiral—and even that adds to how awful you feel.

I believe, from my own experience, that you have to do something active to break that spiral. You can't break it just by thinking more or by telling yourself to relax or change.

I think when people are first told that yoga—or any exercise, for that matter—can help a mood disorder, they don't believe it. This is because very few people talk about sadness and anxiety as if they are illnesses or symptoms, rather than states of being. But sadness and anxiety are transitory. In other words, you can simply find methods to let the feelings go if you're doing something that engages both your mind and your body, as yoga does.

Dean Ornish, a well-known heart disease expert, has found that it is the mind-body connection of yogic exercise that does a body good. The breath work reduces anxiety and perceived stress, which reduces heart rate and blood pressure. The poses improve posture and increase static strength and flexibility, which improve self-confidence and self-image. The meditation aspect increases relaxation and decreases tension.

When you practice yoga, the experts say, you lower the point at which your central nervous system becomes aroused. There is a corresponding reduction in the frequency of panic episodes and a reduced physiological and psychological response to threat.

A study done by Dr. Amparo Castillo-Richmond and the University of California at Los Angeles found that meditation can even reduce the fatty buildup in artery walls. Based on this, many experts extrapolate that if meditation can have a positive effect on heart disease, it can most likely have a positive effect on other health problems, too—especially those, like heart disease, that are stress-related. Another study has shown that people who do yoga are more relaxed and have a more positive attitude than others.

Yoga includes many elements—breathing, meditation, spiritual work, and, of course, the poses. It is the combination of all of these that gives it its confirmed status as a cure-all for depression and anxiety.

Other Helpful Solutions

I'm not a doctor and I can't give medical advice, but I can tell you from my own experience that someone can practice yoga all the time and, if they have severe depression or are struggling with a big issue, they might also need medication, someone to talk with, or a combination of any of the following recommended solutions to overcome it.

Depression and anxiety are both highly treatable, with more than 80 percent of those who seek treatment showing improvement. The earlier treatment begins, the more effective it is and the greater the likelihood of preventing serious recurrences. In trying different modes of treatment, it is important that you accept the idea that your brain is flesh and blood like the rest of your body, and therefore it will respond to lifestyle measures you take to strengthen it.

Some of the most common treatments for depression and anxiety are:

TALK THERAPY. The two types of talk therapy most often prescribed are Behavior Therapy and Cognitive Therapy. Behavior Therapy aims to modify and gain control over unwanted behavior. For example, if a person is afraid of social situations, her therapist might offer her suggestions on what to do at parties and offer support as she attends more get-togethers with lots of people. This kind of therapy gives the individual a sense of control over her life.

The goal of Cognitive Therapy is to change unproductive or harmful thought patterns. The woman in the example above might examine her fears and feelings. She can learn to separate her realistic fears ("I won't have anyone to talk to") from her unrealistic thoughts ("No one likes me and no one ever will"). As with

Behavior Therapy, the individual is actively involved in his or her own recovery and has a sense of control.

Talk therapy helped me at different times in my life because I've needed someone to listen to what has happened and validate my experience and point of view. Talking through my experiences and problems with a supportive and understanding person helped me grow up and learn from, rather than ruminate on, some of the ways I've been treated and some of the things I experienced as a child and teenager.

I've also worked with cognitive therapists. Cognitive therapists help you change the way you think about yourself and your experiences, believing that this will help the way you feel. For example, if you think: "I'm ugly," there's a good chance you'll end up feeling sad and hopeless, which of course is a sign of depression. If, on the other hand, you can think to yourself, "I don't like the way I look in this dress," then you are giving yourself some options (you can take off the dress, you can tell yourself you look better in other outfits) and you aren't left feeling sad.

Behavioral therapists help people with anxiety and nervousness. Let's say, for example, that you get nervous on first dates. A behavioral therapist might have you practice being on a date so that you feel more relaxed when it actually happens. Or, if you are truly having anxiety attacks, both behavioral and cognitive therapists will be able to offer you skills that will help you cope with the symptoms of the attacks.

Most therapists are trained in a number of different styles and will work with you to help you reach your goal, whether it's conquering depression, easing anxiety, or working through parts of your life or personality that you find challenging.

These are a lay-person's view of therapy. I have found therapy to be very help-ful, but I like to think that one reason therapy has worked for me is that I usually go in to see a therapist with a very specific goal. Just as you go to see a dentist because a specific tooth hurts or because you need a cleaning, I believe that ther-apy works when the patient is clear about what she wants (to improve her body image, for example, or to resolve her feelings about a traumatic experience) and understands that it is her responsibility to make that happen, not the therapist's responsibility to "cure" her.

Another form of talk therapy uses relaxation techniques to help people cope effectively with the stresses that contribute to anxiety, as well as with some of the physical symptoms of anxiety. The techniques taught include breath re-training and meditation. Don't be surprised if a therapist suggests you take a yoga class—many Western doctors and therapists now include yogic types of exercises in their treatment of anxiety and depression.

MEDICATION. New and successful medicines are helping sufferers of depression and anxiety. I took Prozac during my severe depression and I honestly believe it saved my life. I do not think I could ever have gotten out of the depth of those feel-ings without medication. However, I will also tell you that my doctor put me on a fairly high dosage, and when I wasn't able to sleep, he wanted to give me a pre-scription for sleeping pills. "Um, I don't want to go on more medication," I told him, "I want to take less. I want to take none, eventually."

With that, my doctor agreed to actually lower my dosage, rather than prescribe another pill. This allowed me to sleep. Four months later, I was off the medication entirely (but still seeing a therapist and, of course, still practicing yoga).

It is amazing to me that my doctor was completely willing to medicate me more before offering me a solution that didn't involve medicine. (Although many of you, I'm sure, won't be as naive as I was about this.) My point in telling you this story is that you shouldn't be afraid of medicine, but you should also know that you need to be an educated consumer. If you don't like the way your doctor is handing out those pills, ask questions and remember—you can always get a second opinion.

EXERCISE. Obviously I believe yoga is a wonderful workout, but I am also a big proponent of a few other forms of exercise. As a certified personal trainer, I can assure you that almost all forms of exercise (except heavy weight lifting) have been shown to relieve depression and anxiety. This includes swimming, walking, and light weight training. Although it's sometimes tough to get active when you're in the throes of despair, I can't encourage you enough to take a walk or go for a swim. Or, of course, do some yoga.

NUTRITION. What and how much you eat has a significant impact on how you feel. Depressed people are usually found to be deficient in specific nutrients, usually many of the B vitamins, fatty acids, and certain minerals. I had been a vegetarian for over 20 years, but when I became severely depressed I started to crave—for the first time in my life—fish. And I started to eat it, too—stunning my family, who had watched me shun all forms of meat since my early teens.

Diets rich in nutrients, rather than high-calorie but nutrient-deficient diets (such as those filled with processed foods and high amounts of sugar) have been shown to contribute to many illnesses, including depression, anxiety, PMS, heart disease, and many cancers. My best advice, without giving you a personalized eating plan, is to eat whole, unprocessed foods as much as possible. Minimize your caffeine intake (especially if you suffer from anxiety) and strive to eat as many fruits, vegetables, whole grains (rather than white flours), and fish as possible.

LIGHT. Even the happiest of us often feel sadder during the short hours of winter daylight than we do during the long, sunny days of summer. If you find yourself oversleeping and craving sweets (a mood lifter) during the winter, you might be light sensitive. If so, one surefire cure is early morning light. Wake up with the sun and get outside—indoor lighting isn't nearly as cheer-inducing as sunlight.

SPIRITUALITY. A deep belief in God—no matter how you envision that entity—has been shown to have a healing effect on people. A connection to the universe and a belief that your life matters can, as seems obvious, prevent you from feeling a sense of worthlessness or hopelessness. I believe that we all need to find our spirituality on our own, and I'm certainly not here to preach, but I will tell you that I honor my Jewish heritage, I practice Buddhism, and I go to Baptist churches with good gospel choirs whenever possible. For me, it's not the religion that matters as much as sharing a life-affirming belief with others who recognize our connection to the universe and our role in it.

FRIENDS. Speaking of sharing with others, people with strong social connections are less likely to suffer from mood disorders. Of course, this can be somewhat of a vicious cycle: If you feel sad and anxious, you're more likely to behave in ways that isolate you from others, thereby hurting your chances of forming lasting friendships. At the same time, when you feel (or truly are) isolated, it's difficult to be more social. Nevertheless, offering friendship to people will help your mood by offering proof that you have value. Sometimes something as simple as making plans to go to a movie with someone can keep a depressed person looking forward to the future. Don't put pressure on yourself to make and have friends, though, because pressure certainly doesn't cheer anyone up. But if you do have friends, stay in touch with them and don't isolate yourself, especially if you're already feeling sad.

LOW-STRESS JOBS. Speaking of pressure brings us to the subject of work. I've always had jobs that were, to a certain extent, challenging. Every couple of years I moved up the corporate ladder and found myself having to learn a new set of skills. When I got sick with depression, I stepped off that corporate ladder for ten months—and man, I loved it! I worked at gyms (teaching yoga and personal training) and I wrote newspaper articles on the fluffiest subjects imaginable. When I look back at that time, I can't tell you how much that little vacation meant to me. I just had so much energy and time to do things that I genuinely enjoyed, rather than working as hard and as often as I used to (and do today).

Having said that, I should also mention that having a job that doesn't challenge you or that offers you no control over your life has also been shown to be a major stress-inducer. If this situation sounds more like yours than mine did, I strongly encourage you to spend some time learning a new skill or getting a job that you enjoy and that values your skills. These things have been shown to greatly contribute to life satisfaction.

HELPING OTHERS. While we shouldn't compare ourselves with others, especially as a way of helping us appreciate our lives and our opportunities, I will say that there is no better way to get out of your own overindulgence in negative thoughts and nervousness than to offer yourself to others. This is especially true if you try to help those who not only need the help, but who also might benefit from some special skill that you have.

In the end, I believe that one of the most important sources of healing is your own intuition. You, more than anyone else, know what will bring happiness into your life. Whether it's getting outside to play tennis more often, teaching a child how to read, or eating a healthy breakfast rather than two doughnuts and a cup of coffee, taking small steps toward health can only do your body and your mind good.

This Yoga Workout

Many people new to yoga assume that the only thing they'll be doing is sitting in Lotus and chanting. But that's not what this yoga workout—or most yoga workouts—are like. Instead we'll be moving pretty actively through numerous poses and using meditation as a tool, but not as the primary focus of our workout.

"Yoga," which in Sanskrit means "union," usually comprises several things: poses, meditation, breathing exercises, and, although they aren't covered in this book, eating choices (such as vegetarianism) and spiritual decisions (such as nonviolence).

I have studied yoga through books and videos and with teachers in four different states. I have taught yoga to beginners through advanced students. I think

WHAT IS "MOVING THROUGH"?

There are two ways to practice yoga poses. You can get into a pose and hold it for a particular period of time, such as 10 breath cycles or one minute. Iyengar practitioners do this, building longer time periods and more intense stretches into each pose (the longer you hold the pose, the more deeply you can get into it), but also allowing for rest periods in between poses.

Other yogis, such as those who practice Astanga and Vinyasa yoga, get into each pose very deeply but don't hold it for as long. Instead, they "flow" from one pose to the next. Their practice consists of not just taking each pose to its limit, but also in flowing fluidly and intensely from one pose to the next. This creates more of a "cardio" workout—your heart rate goes up because you're active throughout the session.

One style of yoga isn't better than the other. There are benefits to each, and I find both types of classes enjoyable. The programs in this book feature both yoga styles. In order to facilitate the flow style of yoga, I've included a section called "Moving Through" in those chapters. There you'll find instructions on how to link the poses together in a flowing sequence. However, you don't have to do this. Each of the poses works on its own, and you should feel free to do one pose at a time, especially when you are first learning them. As I've said (and will probably say again), there is no one right way to do yoga. As long as you read the instructions for each pose carefully so you avoid moving in an awkward manner, you should feel free to practice any pose wherever and whenever you want.

I've taken a class in just about every type of yoga available, including Iyengar, Kripalu, Astanga, Bikram, Kundalini, Sivinanda, and Vinyasa. I like all of them, so I've used elements from most of these forms when coming up with these pose prescriptions.

This workout incorporates elements from my study of Bikram yoga, which was created by Bikram Choudhury and features a series of 26 poses. Classes in this style are always conducted in a studio that is kept at around 100°F, which is why it is often referred to as "hot" yoga. I've also studied Astanga yoga, which features a series of strenuous poses that are done quickly and in a flowing fashion. The Iyengar and Sivinanda styles of yoga are the types most of us first practice when learning yoga. In it, poses are held for a longer period than in the two previously mentioned styles and students often rest between poses.

Kundalini yoga is lots of fun, raising the energy through breathing, sound, and hand positions. Viniyasa stresses the use of postures, as well as breath, meditation, ritual, and prayer. I value its teachings because I believe, as many yogis do, that yoga isn't about the physical knowledge you can gain but the spiritual and life practices you can adopt.

I want to reassure you that the history of yoga is vague in many ways, and you do not have to change religions, dress differently, or get a new group of vegetarian friends in order to practice yoga or do this workout. All you have to do is open your mind to the possibility that yoga may help you feel better. That's it.

As you probably know, many of the postures you will see in this book have Sanskrit names, just as the word "yoga" itself is Sanskrit. But because those names have changed over the years and because the Sanskrit names are

SOME YOGA TIPS

Even though yoga is a holistic mind-body experience, there are a few tricks to doing it "right." I put that word in quotation marks, because I want to reiterate that there's no such thing as "wrong" yoga, except the kind that forces people to do more than they are able to in an effort to do the pose "right."

Nevertheless, there are ways to be more successful at holding poses longer or getting your posture to be more precise. Here are some general yoga tips.

▶ When balancing, focus on something outside of your body, such as a spot on the wall or floor, and don't worry about falling over—you won't. Focus on keeping your entire foot on the floor and let your body flow with your breath, rather than forcing it to be "still."

▶ Don't wear socks or sneakers; be barefoot. This is important for two reasons. One, your entire foot needs to flatten on the floor in order to balance properly, and two, your brain actually "listens" to your feet and ankles in order to balance properly. This is called "proprioception," and your balance will improve faster and better if you give those special spots (called proprioceptors) in your feet and ankles the chance to "talk" to your brain. Your body will create a more complete and useful muscle memory of standing properly if your feet are bare.

▶ Wear clothes that are comfortable and easy to move in. Our model uses tight clothing so that you can see the pose clearly, but it's important to wear loose clothes when possible. And, if you're pressed for time, don't even worry about wearing the "right" clothes. I do my morning yoga in my pajamas or nightgown and my evening yoga in pajama pants and a tank top. At work? I've been known to go into Downward Facing Dog wearing a skirt and tights.

▶ If you're doing yoga early in the day, such as the morning routine, give yourself a minute to warm up before starting. Have a glass of water or some tea, move around a little, and then expect your first few sun salutations to be a little "sticky," meaning you won't be able to flex as much as usual or hold the poses for very long. Your body needs time to warm up.

▶ It is preferable to do yoga in a warm room. Bikram is done in a very warm room, around 100°F, and many students wear bathing suits to let their skin breathe. It feels great, but you won't want to heat a room in your house to that temperature. Instead, make sure your room is at least 68° to 70°F so that your muscles stay warm and pliable. If your room isn't warm, pile on loose clothes.

▶ Always have a bottle or glass of water nearby. You may not sweat during this workout like you do during a cardio session at the gym, but you need to be well hydrated during any exercise.

meaningless to me (and hard to pronounce), I'm simply using the English names I've heard in my various classes. If you study with another teacher or even read another book, you may see these poses under various names. Don't worry about it—that's the nature of yoga and its long history.

What makes something "yoga"—whether it's a push-up-style pose or a Downward Facing Dog—is the intention with which the pose is practiced. You should bring to your yoga practice awareness, a calming breath, and the intention to let negative energy out of your body. The intention of a push-up in yoga is not to get great pecs so you can look good in a tank top. Instead, the intention is to gather your energy, use it wisely, and center yourself. Yoga asks you to let yourself become the pose, rather than remain a depressed or anxious person looking for an answer.

Finally, yoga asks that you not worry about doing a pose perfectly. It asks that you not say to yourself, "I will be happy when I achieve a perfect backbend or when I look better in my new yoga outfit." Happiness and serenity cannot be postponed. Instead, yoga—in the form of exercises and meditation as a spiritual practice—asks that you be serene and peaceful in this very moment.

What Are "Modifications, Variations, and Props?"

After each pose I describe in this book, there is a section called "Modifications, Variations, and Props." Most yoga poses have a long list of modifications and variations that enable anyone, at any ability level, to do a pose in his or her own way.

I don't necessarily present the easiest or the hardest versions of each pose in this book, but I do offer as many variations as possible for all levels of students.

Likewise, in an effort to make yoga accessible to all students, many yogis use common props that assist people in reaching certain postures.

BLANKETS. Used to support the body during restorative (restful) poses and to cover the body for warmth during meditation and breathing practice, yoga blankets are usually made of wool. They fold easily and stay rather firm in order to bolster the body securely. You can use any type of blanket as a support, but most comforters don't have enough weight to hold the body. You should be able to feel the support of a blanket, not sink into it if you lie on top of it.

BLOCKS. Some yoga poses require you to, for example, bend forward from the waist and touch your fingers to the floor. If you can't reach that far, you can put a block on the floor and rest your hands on that. This allows you to move into the pose completely but not force yourself into a position that is uncomfortable or potentially dangerous. Blocks are typically made of foam and measure about 9 x 5 $^1/_2$ x 3 $^1/_2$ inches. You can use them in any direction, giving yourself 9 inches of length or just a small boost of 3 $^1/_2$ inches. You can also rest your weight on the blocks, as they are strong and can support the body.

CHAIRS, BALLS, AND BACK PROPS. An open-backed chair or a large exercise ball allows you to go into backbend, for example, without having to support your body. The support helps create a restful pose while still engaging your muscles and extending the stretch.

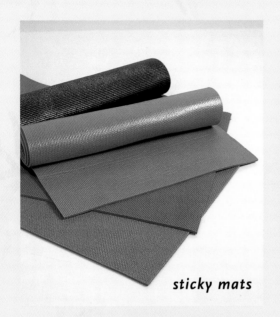

sticky mats

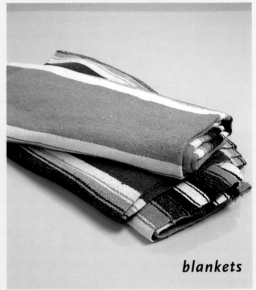

blankets

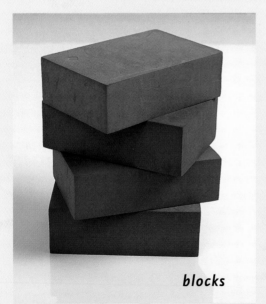

blocks

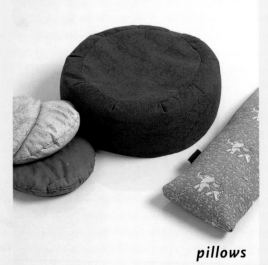

pillows

STICKY MATS. New yoga students are often quick to judge themselves when it comes to balancing. "Why can't I stay on one foot?" they ask themselves. Well, frequently it's more about the floor they're standing on than their balancing skills. Wood floors are excellent for yoga, but sometimes your feet (and your back and butt, during floor and sitting postures) benefit from a little cushioning, which these mats provide.

PILLOWS. Yogis use both eye pillows and regular bed pillows in their practice. Eye pillows go, as the name suggests, over your eyes to increase the sense of restfulness and keep out light during meditation. Their weight (they are usually filled with scented buckwheat shells) forces the muscles around the eyes to relax, decreasing tension in the face.

You can also use firm bed pillows for support during many poses. Although this isn't a traditional way to do yoga, I have found that many regular pillows are firmer than blankets and thus provide more support during backbends and other poses that are sometimes done with props.

STRAPS. Less-flexible people often use straps to extend a stretch. For instance, you can wrap a strap around your foot during leg stretches in order to pull your leg that much closer to your torso.

Wherever possible, I have made suggestions for props in the description of each pose, but you shouldn't feel compelled to use them. Some people are helped by the props, while others prefer to work without them. Experiment to see what works for you.

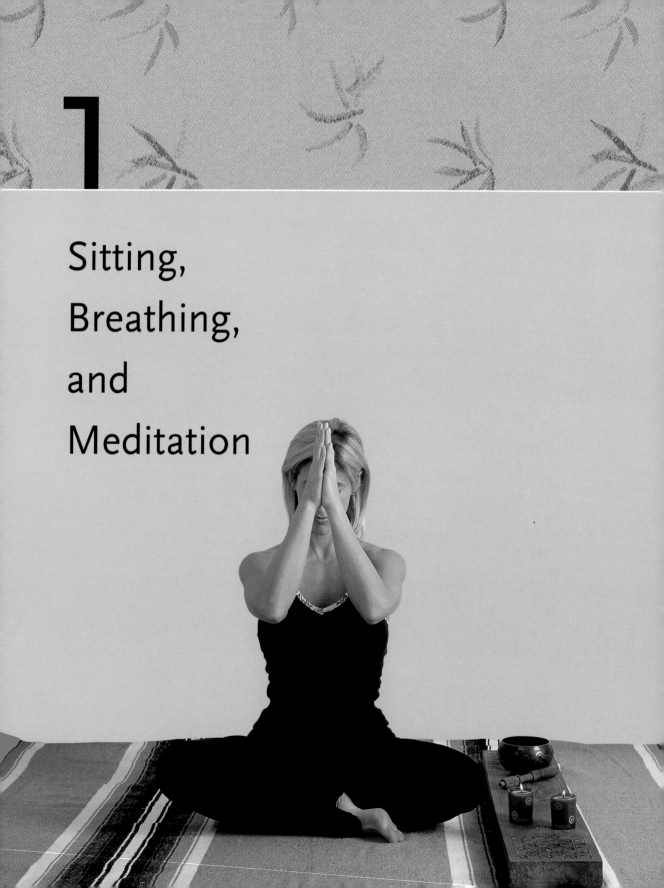

1

Sitting, Breathing, and Meditation

"When all else fails, sit quietly and breathe consciously."

—ANONYMOUS

THIS IS ONE OF MY FAVORITE YOGA QUOTES. IT'S A BRILLIANT PIECE OF ADVICE, BECAUSE WHEN confronted with a problem, most of us feel a need to "do" something. We want to talk, we want to confront, and we want to fix whatever's wrong. Also, when we are upset or bothered, our emotions take over and our thinking goes out the window. That loss of serenity can lead our bodies into a dark, unhappy place. Our stomachs get upset, and we may feel our nervous system get agitated and ready to defend ourselves, or even to attack.

Sitting quietly and breathing consciously contradicts both of those actions. If we are quiet, we cannot speak and make the problem worse. If we are breathing consciously, our nervous system relaxes and we are better able to soothe ourselves. In fact, we are soothing ourselves.

Of course, it is difficult to sit quietly, and it is especially difficult when we are upset and depressed. When I was depressed, sitting quietly was almost impossible for me: I was always on the phone, always repeating the same concerns and fears to my friends over and over again. But over time I was able to learn to sit with my feelings and, more than that, to let them go and be.

Proper breathing and conscious thought make up yoga's easy two-step plan for reaching a state of loving kindness. But first, I need to teach you how to sit.

Sitting

I bet you're thinking that sitting, like walking, breathing, and sleeping, is something you already know how to do. And you do. I don't want you to start feeling self-conscious and I also want to reassure you right up front that you can breathe properly and meditate anywhere and anytime. Nevertheless, when you connect breathing and meditation with sitting properly, you create a completely healing experience. It engages your body in connection with your spirit, thus setting the scene for true relaxation. But more than all of these reasons, I believe that creating a specific place and manner to sit, breathe, and meditate encourages an intention toward peace of mind.

There are three sitting postures in this book (see Lotus, Hero, and Cobbler on page 37). Each works fine for meditation. I would encourage you to try each of these postures when you meditate and practice your breathing so that you can find the one that is most relaxing to you.

White Light Meditation

If you're down in the dumps right now, it's likely that you rarely speak to yourself with love and kindness. For years I lived with a voice inside my head that constantly criticized everything I did and who I was. "There's no way someone will ever love you. You should be more successful by now. You weigh too much." On and on I would go, never saying anything supportive or loving to myself.

As I write this, my son is almost three years old. All day, every day that I spend with him, I consistently encourage him with love and kindness. If he spills something, I tell him it's not important and that he's doing a good job learning how

Lotus

Hero

Cobbler

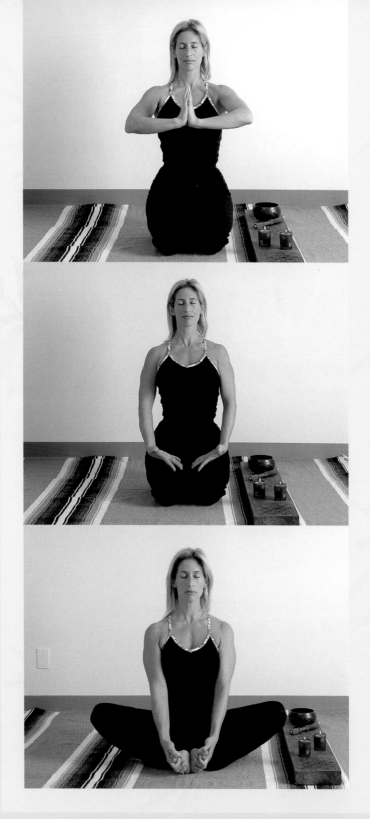

to hold a cup. If I can't understand what he's trying to say to me, I tell him that I love him and that I want to help him, and that if he slows down and speaks more slowly, I'll do my best to understand. Even when he does something naughty on purpose, such as snatching a toy from a friend, and I have to reprimand his behavior, I focus my displeasure on what he did, not who he is, and I remind him that he is a good person who can learn how to behave properly. In other words, I accept my son for who he is. I love him unconditionally, and I trust that he is doing the very best he can do.

I can tell you right now that while it doesn't take any effort for me to nurture my child, it is a huge effort—like Sisyphus pushing the boulder up the hill—for me to learn to nurture and love myself. For years my friends and family told me that I was too hard on myself. I didn't even understand how they could say something like that. Didn't they see how awful I was? Didn't they understand how much punishment I deserved?

This kind of thinking can only lead to depression. Who can be happy when someone is running them down all day? You cannot thrive in an unkind environment. Fortunately, yoga can help you silence your inner critic and teach you to speak to yourself in a more loving manner. But I will tell you that it is almost impossible to simply expect that you can tell yourself to stop saying nasty things to yourself and be nice. That would be somewhat like telling yourself to lose 10 pounds without figuring out how to eat differently and exercise more.

I've taught this meditation to hundreds of people. This meditation works for me because it reminds me that what I need is right inside me at all times. When you're depressed, it's easy to believe that you will feel better when something outside of yourself happens—when you get a boyfriend, when you have more money, when you lose 10 pounds. But that's not true. What you need, just like Dorothy said, just like every wise person says, is right here, right now.

The concept of "white light" stems from chakras, which many yogis believe are the eight energy centers throughout the body that correspond to specific emotions, bodily functions, and colors. The eighth chakra is white and surrounds the body. Kundalini yogis believe that this energy field can grow brighter and larger through yoga and meditation.

Even if this concept seems foreign to you, remember that many Christian artists depict angels and other heavenly beings with a field of white light around them. Halos are a form of white light. I choose to imagine that this bright white light is a visual metaphor for a peaceful, blissful state—and I believe that it is possible for all of us to achieve it. For our purposes, the white light in this meditation symbolizes your divine spirit, whatever that means to you.

You'll have to read the following meditation over a few times so you'll remember it and be able to think through it while you sit and breathe fully. Please remember that although I use the words "inhale" and "exhale" throughout the meditation, those are only cues and reminders to breathe deeply and fully. You don't have to breathe only where those words are written.

Finally, I would like to encourage you to either record this meditation to listen to it while you sit or to have someone read it to you as you sit. Being receptive, rather than active, during a meditation is truly restful. More than that, though, restfulness allows your brain to absorb the message more fully. It's almost like learning the lyrics to a song by listening to it over and over.

Sit comfortably, place your hands in a position that you find comfortable, and if possible, make the room slightly dark. (You don't want the room pitch black so you don't fall asleep or become disoriented when you're finished.)

Close your eyes.

Inhale. Bring your breath in through your nose and feel it fill up the space behind your face, in your head, and down your throat and neck. Feel the air drift down into your shoulders and chest. Let the air fill up your torso and your abdomen. Feel it go into your hips and thighs. The air is moving down your legs, into your calves and feet. Feel it fill your toes.

Now, when you exhale, let the air drift out of your mouth and over your lips. Feel everything sink a little as the air leaves your body. Let the air go.

On your next inhalation, as you bring the air in through your nose, I want you to imagine that a bright white light is coming in with the air. Feel the air and the white light fill up the space behind your face, in your head, and down your throat and neck. Feel the white light and the oxygen drift down into your shoulders and chest. Let the air and white light fill up your torso and your abdomen. Feel it go into your hips and thighs. The air and the white light are moving down your legs, into your calves and feet. Feel your toes fill with air and light.

Now, on your next exhalation, you're going to let the air go and feel your body sink, but you'll keep the white light inside you. There's nothing magical or mystical about this white light. It is always inside you, keeping you warm, safe, and happy. So let the air go, but keep the white light.

On your next inhalation, I want you to bring the air in and feel it fill the white light, making it so white and so bright that it pushes out of your body and surrounds you. Feel the air and the white light surround your face, head, throat, and neck. Feel the air and white light surround your shoulders and chest. Let the air fill up your torso and your abdomen as the white light covers your belly and back. Feel the white light surround your hips and thighs. The air is moving down your legs, into your calves and feet as the white light surrounds your lower body. Feel the air fill your toes as the white light envelops the rest of your body.

On your next exhalation, as you let the air go, keep the white light inside you and around you. You don't have to tell people about this white light; they will sense that you feel calm, happy, and safe. So let the air go, but keep the white light.

Inhale again, bringing the air in to make the white light even brighter and whiter. Then let the air go, keeping the white light.

Continue to do this until you are ready to open your eyes, feeling more centered, balanced, and calmer.

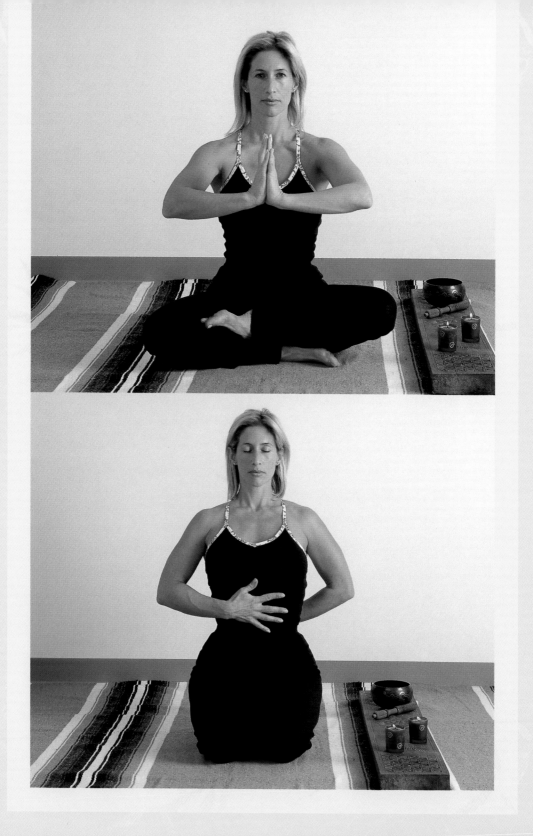

Breathing

One of the most genius aspects of breathing consciously is that once you learn to do it in a sitting pose—whether it's cross-legged or full lotus—you can take that knowledge and apply it to your active yoga practice. You will have the ability to breathe deeply no matter how active your body is. Even if you're in the midst of a fully loaded Astanga routine, for example, you will still be able to breathe deeply and practice your poses without losing your breath or even becoming winded.

Yoga breathing is a Western phrase that corresponds to the Sanskrit word *pranayama*. *Prana* means the breath or life force and *yama* is the motion of breathing. During my first class with any yoga students, I spend a few minutes helping everyone unlearn their idea of a "deep breath." Very often our idea of a "deep breath" is one in which we gasp as much air as possible and grab onto it in the very top of our lungs, holding it, holding it, holding it, until we are forced to let it go. This is not good breathing.

Pranayama is the ability to breathe in a calm, smooth, effective manner. To do this, I want you to sit comfortably; don't worry about your posture. You'll obviously have to read through this a few times as you practice, but eventually I hope you'll be able to close your eyes to breathe properly.

Close your mouth gently and inhale through your nose in a very calm and relaxed fashion. Don't rush, and don't try to bring as much air as possible into your body. Instead, I want you to focus on bringing your breath down through your nose, down your throat, and into your chest, filling up your lungs completely and then filling deep into your belly. Don't try to hold your breath—just coax it along, visualizing it filling up your torso. While you do this you can hold your hands over your heart center in Prayer pose, or you can place one hand on your stomach and one on your back so you can feel your whole torso expanding with each breath.

Hold your breath for just a second and then, just as gently and calmly as you inhaled, let the air float out of your nose (or if you are more comfortable, through your mouth).

That was a deep breath.

Did you notice that nothing intense happened? Did you notice, too, that your breath probably took a little longer to travel into your lungs than it usually does? Your lungs expand in all directions—up, down, forward, and to the sides. A deep breath means that you fill your lungs and send that air through your body, feeding it with as much oxygen as you can give it.

The focus you just gave to your breath is what we mean by breathing "consciously." You were in the moment. Your activity was breathing and your mind was engaged in what your body was doing.

Picture a person driving her car and talking on her cell phone. Which activity is she conscious of? Probably neither. Consciousness doesn't refer to a hyper-awareness of a moment—you aren't thinking deeply about breathing or wondering what philosophical implications a deep breath has. You are simply mindfully aware of what you body is doing and, in this case, it is breathing.

Putting It All Together

You may be tempted to say that you sit, breathe, and tell yourself to relax everyday, and still you've got the blues. I can only reassure you that proper sitting, intentional breathing, and conscious meditation are as different from the kind of sitting most of us do on a daily basis as ballet dancing is from slipping on a banana.

It may seem like a lot to remember, but these three elements go together naturally and, if you practice each one on its own one or two times, when you bring it all together you will find that the whole is truly more than the sum of its parts.

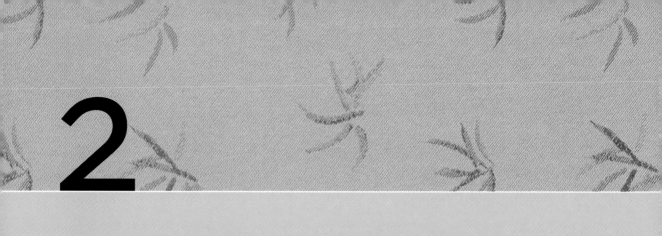

2

Morning Routine to Wake Up and Energize for the Day

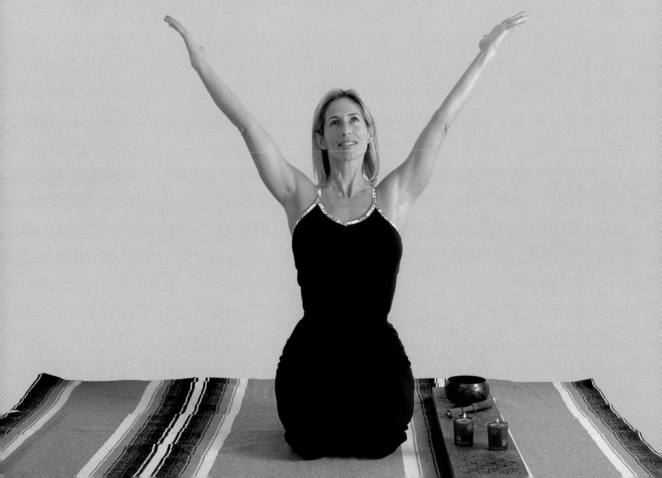

MORNING IS TOUGH FOR DEPRESSED PEOPLE. ONE OF THE MOST TELLING PHYSICAL SYMPTOMS of depression is waking up very early (in the middle of the night, really—the dark 3 A.M. of the soul, as F. Scott Fitzgerald called it), and then, of course, after lying in bed worrying or obsessing or feeling sad for a few hours, maybe you fall back asleep at 5 or 7 A.M., and that whole cycle of sleeping, obsessing, and sleeping some more starts the day off badly.

I've found that there are two guarantees for a good night's sleep. The first is having something to look forward to upon waking up. Although it can be a tough habit to get into, going to sleep with a goal for the next day and doing all you can to simply reach that goal is a great first step toward feeling more hopeful about the next day. In this chapter, I will teach you the Sun Salutation, a sequence of poses that will wake you up and make you feel great from the very start of your day, as well as give you something to look forward to from the time you go to bed at night.

(In case you're wondering, the second step to getting a good night's sleep is creating the right atmosphere for rest, and I talk about that in Chapter 6 beginning on page 127.)

Each step of the Sun Salutation is a pose unto itself, so if you can't do them all in a row, you're still doing yoga if you just do one pose, rather than the whole series. Each pose, as you will see, has its own list of benefits.

Moving Through

This is a series of 14 poses that flow together seamlessly. Once you become comfortable with each pose, you will be able to move from one into the next in such a way that even the motion between the poses will help you energize and relax.

You should do the Sun Salutation at least six times, alternating with each leg three times (this will make sense as you read through the following instructions). Breathe purposefully and consistently throughout the motion, and form the intention to go fully into each pose.

Do not rush through the poses. You will not gain any physical benefit by going quickly. The benefit truly comes from feeling strong and moving your body in an intense, elegant manner, whether you're in a pose or between poses.

Each pose is explained in more detail following these instructions.

1. Begin in Mountain pose. Inhale, bring your arms out to your sides and then up and over your head. Arch back, pushing your hips forward. Do not drop your head down by crunching your neck. Instead, stretch your neck and upper back up and over an imaginary arch. (Think of making the same shape as the Nike swoosh.)

2. Exhale and dive slowly into Forward Bend. When moving from Mountain to Forward Bend, you can either keep your hands and arms out to your sides or you can keep them raised above your head. Once in Forward Bend, bring your hands to the floor if possible. If not, bring them to your feet, ankles, or shins Do not pull

yourself into a deeper bend. Instead, let your inhalation and exhalation move your upper body down and closer to your legs.

3. Inhale, keeping your hands on the floor or your legs or feet, while you straighten your back and bring your head up and away from your legs. Keep your eyes forward and straighten your neck to help elongate your back. Your shape should be very angular—one straight line from your heels to your butt and then a perpendicular straight line from your butt to the crown of your head.

4. Exhale and return to forward bend, feeling yourself go deeper into the pose.

5. Inhale and lunge back with your right leg. The bottom of your right foot should face up (so you're resting on the front of your lower right leg and the top of your right foot). Keep your right leg straight and strong, pushing your hips forward in the lunge. (You should feel a stretch in the front of your right thigh and make sure that your right knee is over—but not past—the toes of your right foot.) At the same time, arch your back "over the sun," raising your arms above you and back. Keep your neck in an elegant line with your back, and pull your shoulders down. If this is too difficult, simply rest your hands on your bent left leg while maintaining your balance.

6. Exhale, bring your hands to the ground in front of you, and bring your left leg back to meet your right. Turn your toes under and come down, slowly, into Plank pose. Keep your elbows close to your sides, your neck aligned with your back, and your eyes looking forward.

7. Inhale as you roll over your toes and come into Cobra. The top of your feet should be against the floor as you arch the upper part of your torso and head up.

8. Exhale as you press up into Downward Facing Dog pose. Press your upper body through your arms and lift your hips.

9. Inhale, return to the Lunge, this time with your right leg forward. Arch back over the sun. Make sure your right foot is as far forward as possible, but that your knee isn't going past your toes.

10. Exhale, put your hands on the ground, and come up into Forward Bend.

11. Inhale, straighten your back and look forward.

12. Exhale, return to Forward Bend.

13. Inhale, extend your arms out to the sides while you come up to Mountain.

14. Exhale, as you bring your hands into Prayer position, palms pressed gently together, just in front of your heart.

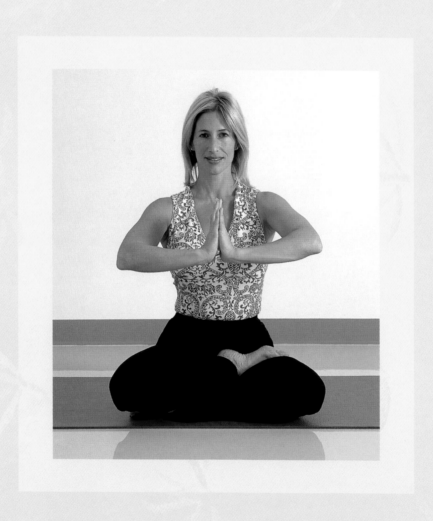

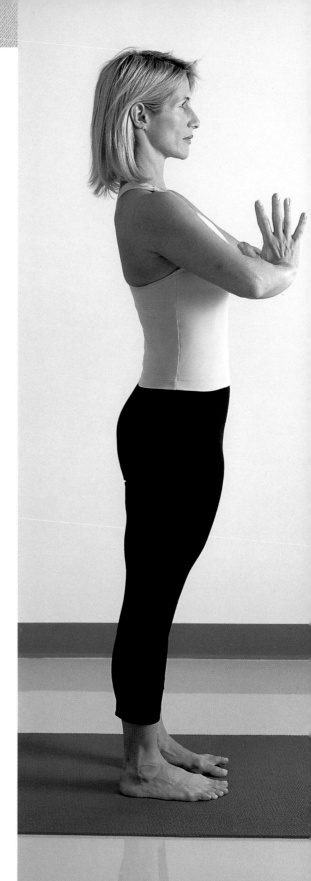

Mountain

Mountain is simply the perfect standing position—whether you're doing yoga or standing in line at the grocery store. Once you begin to stand properly in yoga class, you'll carry this skill into the rest of your life. Good posture is part of the mind-body link: When you stand up properly, your lungs have more room to breathe fully; your spine is supported, taking away small aches and pains; and you feel free to move gracefully.

1 Stand with your big toes touching, heels slightly apart, feet parallel. Rock back and forth and side to side. Gradually reduce this swaying to a standstill, with your weight balanced evenly between your feet.

2 Firm your thigh muscles and lift your kneecaps. Bring your hands into prayer position just in front of your chest. Lift your inner ankles to strengthen your inner arches, then imagine a line of energy all the way up along your inner thighs to your groin, and from there through the core of your torso, neck, and head, and out through the crown of your head. Turn your upper thighs slightly inward. Lengthen your tailbone toward the floor and lift your pubis toward your navel.

3 Press your shoulder blades into your back, then widen them across and release them down your back. Without pushing your lower front ribs forward, lift your chest toward the ceiling. Widen your collarbones. Hang your arms beside the torso.

4 Balance the crown of your head directly over the center of your pelvis, with the underside of your chin parallel to the floor, throat soft, and tongue wide and flat on the floor of your mouth. Soften your eyes.

Modifications, Variations, and Props

▶ You can check your alignment in this pose with your back against a wall. Stand with the backs of your heels, sacrum, and shoulder blades (but not the back of your head) touching the wall. Stand straight with your hips tucked under and shoulders down.

▶ You can challenge your balance by practicing this pose with your eyes closed.

▶ You can alter the position of your arms in a variety of ways:

- Hold your hands in Prayer pose, centered in front of your chest,
- Stretch your arms upward, perpendicular to the floor and parallel with each other, with your palms facing inward,
- Interlace your fingers, extend your arms straight out in front of your torso, turn your palms away, and then stretch your arms overhead so your palms face the ceiling,
- Cross your arms behind your back, holding each elbow with the opposite-side hand (be sure to reverse the cross of the forearms and repeat for an equal length of time).

▶ You can improve your balance in this pose by standing with your inner feet anywhere from 3 to 5 inches apart.

Mountain strengthens the entire body, especially the leg, abdominal, and back muscles. It relaxes the shoulder muscles and firms the buttocks.

Standing Forward Bend

New yogis often assume the "point" of this pose is to get your head as close to your legs as possible, but that's not the case. From a physical point of view, your goal in Standing Forward Bend is to maintain good posture, even though you're bent in two. In other words, yoga teachers like to see straight legs (if possible) and flat backs, as well as hips high in the air. From a mental point of view, the point, as in all other postures, is to remain relaxed and breathing deeply throughout the pose.

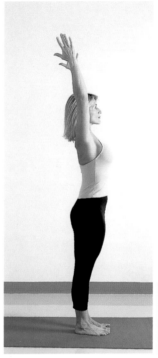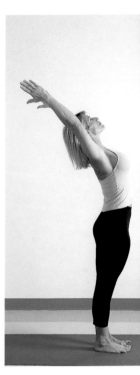

This pose stretches the hamstrings, calves, and hips and strengthens the thighs and knees.

1. Stand in Mountain pose and bring your hands out to your sides and up above your head. Arch your body backward, and then as you exhale, bend forward from your hip joints, not from your waist. As you descend, draw your front torso out of your groin and open the space between your pubis and top sternum. As in all forward bends, the emphasis is on lengthening the front torso as you move more fully into the position.

2. If possible, with your knees straight, bring your palms or fingertips to the floor slightly in front of or beside your feet, or bring your palms to the backs of your ankles. If this isn't possible, cross your forearms and hold your elbows. Press your heels firmly into the floor and lift your sitting bones toward the ceiling. Turn your top thighs slightly inward.

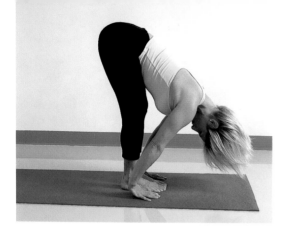

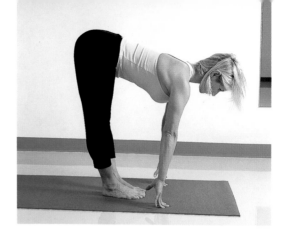

3 With each inhalation in the pose, lift and lengthen your front torso just slightly; with each exhalation release a little more fully into the forward bend. In this way the torso oscillates almost imperceptibly with your breath. As you bend forward, let your head hang from the root of your neck, which is deep in the upper back, between the shoulder blades.

4 After bending forward, slide the index and middle finger of each hand in between the big toe and second toe of each foot. Then curl your fingers under the bottom and around your big toe and wrap your thumb around your fingers. With an inhalation, straighten your arms and lift your front torso away from your thighs, making your back as concave as possible. Hold for a few breaths, then exhale and lengthen down and forward, bending your elbows out to the sides.

Modifications, Variations, and Props

▶ Do this pose with bent knees, or perform it with your hands on a wall, legs perpendicular to your torso, and arms parallel to the floor.

▶ To increase the stretch in the backs of your legs, stand with the balls of your feet elevated an inch or more off the floor on a sand bag or thick book.

▶ If you're performing the pose by itself, don't roll your spine to come up. Instead bring your hands to your hips and stretch your front torso out long. Then press your tailbone down and into your pelvis and come up on an inhalation with a long front torso.

▶ To increase the stretch in the backs of your legs, bend your knees slightly. Imagine that your sacrum is sinking deeper into the back of your pelvis and bring your tailbone closer to your pubis. Against this resistance, push your top thighs back and heels down and straighten your knees again. Be careful not to straighten your knees by locking them back (you can press your hands against the back of each knee to provide some resistance). Instead, let them straighten slowly as you raise your hips.

Bent Knee Lunge/Arms Over the Sun

This is a great all-body stretch that allows you to breathe deeply while you move. This move is also a good warm-up pose for any workout, as it prepares your body for deeper stretches.

1 From the Forward Bend, keep your hands in place on the floor. Step your right foot back as far as possible and bend your left knee, getting into a lunge position. Your left knee should be over your foot, but not past your toes. (You should be able to see your toes if you look down.)

2 Straighten your right leg, keeping the front of your foot and leg down against the floor.

3 Push your hips forward as you release your hands from the floor and bring them up, past the front of your body and over your head. Focus on pressing your right thigh and knee down toward the floor while you're lifting up out of your torso. You should have a real feeling of opposition throughout your entire body: hips pushing forward, legs pressing down, and arms pressing up and back.

4 Be sure to keep your shoulders down and round your spine, as if you're bending back "over the sun," rather than forcing your neck down and toward your back. Your back should make a very rounded C shape as you reach far up with your fingers.

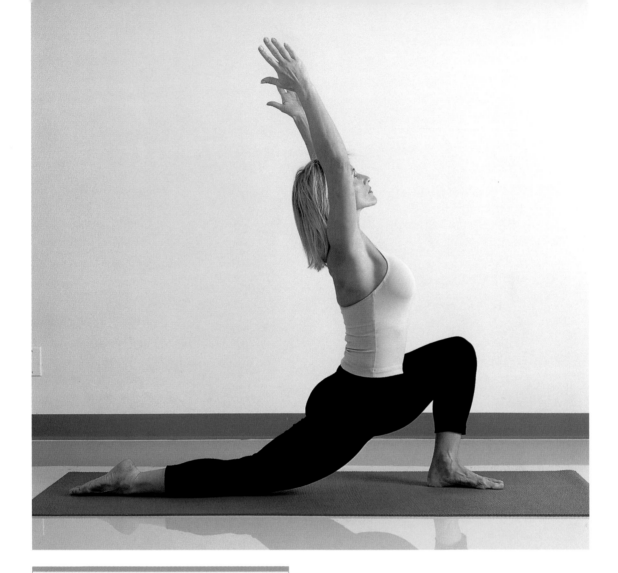

Modifications, Variations, and Props

▶ If you find it difficult to balance in this pose, feel free to keep your hands on the floor or on your bent knee. You can still stretch your spine and shoulders, even though the amount of stretch will be decreased a bit.

▶ You can also keep your straight knee slightly bent, letting just your thigh, knee, and foot touch the floor, rather than the entire leg.

This pose strengthens the back of the body, including the hamstrings, and stretches the front of the body, including the quadriceps, hip flexors, abdominal muscles, pectorals, shoulders, and neck. It increases flexibility and releases tension in the spine. It's a good all-body balancer, as it is done at least twice during any workout, thereby letting each leg stretch and support during a session.

Plank

This is the yoga "push-up." Plank strengthens the entire body, but it is particularly challenging to the core muscles of your torso— the transverse abdominal and back muscles. From a mind-body perspective, Plank asks you to move slowly and with control without sacrificing form.

1 Begin with your hands on the floor, directly under your shoulders. Your toes should be flat on the floor, heels and arches pressed back behind you. Firm your shoulder blades against your back ribs and press your tailbone toward your pubis. Your body should be in a long, diagonal line from your toes to your head. Look down, with the crown of your head facing in front of you and your neck long and relaxed.

2 There's a tendency in this pose to let your lower back sway toward the floor and your tailbone poke up toward the ceiling. Fight this tendency by keeping your tailbone firmly in place and your legs very active and turned slightly inward. Draw your pubis toward your navel. Keep the space between your shoulder blades broad. Don't let your elbows splay out to the sides; hold them close to the sides of your torso and push them back toward your heels. Press the bases of your index fingers firmly into the floor. Lift the top of your sternum and your head to look forward, without bending your neck.

3 With an exhalation, bend your elbows and slowly lower your torso and legs to a few inches above and parallel to the floor. Keep your elbows in toward your sides, shoulders pressed down and back, and your neck long.

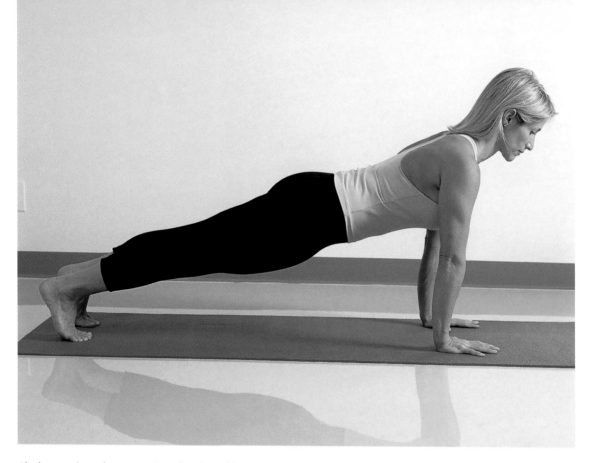

Plank strengthens the arms, wrists, gluteals, and hamstrings. It also tones the abdominal muscles and back.

Modifications, Variations, and Props

▶ You can get a feel for this challenging position by practicing it while facing a wall. Stand a few inches away from the wall and press your hands against it, slightly lower than the level of your shoulders. Imagine that you are trying to push yourself away from the wall, but allow your shoulder blades to prevent the actual movement. Lengthen your tailbone into your heels and lift your sternum toward the ceiling.

▶ Another challenging variation: While performing Plank on the ground, inhale and lift one leg parallel to the floor. Press strongly through your raised heel and lengthen through the crown of your head, keeping your tailbone pressed towards your pubis. Hold for 10 to 30 seconds, exhale your foot to the floor, and then repeat with the other leg for the same length of time.

▶ Open the space between your shoulder blades. As you press your outer arms inward, push your shoulder blades into this resistance. Make sure you don't narrow across the collarbones as you do this.

Cobra

A wonderful stretch for the chest, symbolically bringing joy into your heart, Cobra requires both upper and lower body strength. Its focus on the curve of the back and removes a lot of tension from the body.

1 Lie on your belly on the floor. Stretch your legs back, placing the tops of your feet on the floor. Bend your elbows and spread your palms on the floor beside your waist so that your forearms are relatively perpendicular to the floor. Inhale and press your inner hands firmly into the floor and slightly back, as if you were trying to push yourself forward along the floor.

2 On an inhalation, straighten your arms and lift your torso up and off the floor. Keep your thighs firm and turned slightly inward, your arms firm and turned out so your elbow creases face forward.

3 Press your tailbone toward your pubis and lift your pubis toward your navel. Firm but don't harden your buttocks.

4 Lower your shoulder blades and expand chest and sides. Lift through the top of your sternum, but avoid pushing your chest forward. Look straight ahead or tip your head back slightly, but take care not to compress the back of your neck or harden your throat.

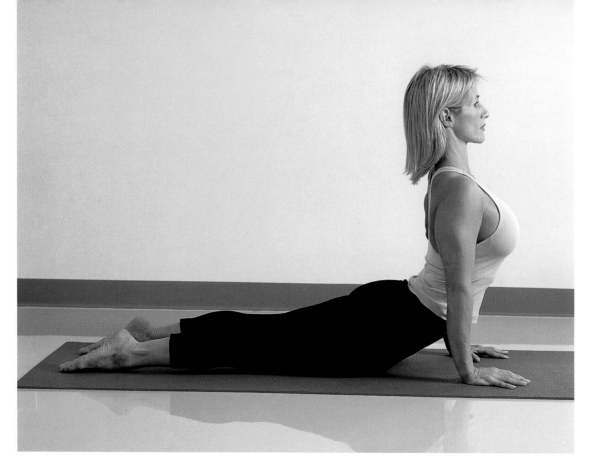

Cobra opens the chest, stretches the shoulders and abdominal muscles, and improves posture. It also strengthens the spine, arms, and wrists, and firms the buttocks.

Modifications, Variations, and Props

▶ You can practice this pose by itself, holding it for anywhere from 15 to 30 seconds while breathing easily. If it's difficult to keep your legs strongly suspended above the floor and you can't remain in the pose for as long as you want to, position a thick blanket roll below your top thighs before you begin the pose. When you are in the pose, lightly rest your thighs on this roll as you press your tailbone closer to the roll.

▶ There's a tendency in this pose to "hang" on your shoulders, which lifts them up toward your ears and crunches your neck. Actively draw your shoulders away from your ears by lengthening down along your sides and pulling your shoulder blades toward your tailbone.

▶ You can also do Upward Facing Dog, a pose similar to Cobra, by pushing off the floor from the tops of your feet and the bottoms of your hands, lifting your legs and lower torso from the floor.

Downward Facing Dog

Possibly everyone's favorite yoga pose, this is the first pose my son learned—as a one-year-old! Downward Facing Dog stretches and strengthens the entire body, releasing tension from every muscle and sore spot. I can't recommend highly enough practicing this pose on its own whenever you feel tense or worried. A partial inversion (part of your body is upside-down), it brings blood to your brain, which can improve your mood while you're working your muscles.

1. Come to your hands and knees on the floor. Place your knees directly below your hips and your hands slightly in front of your shoulders. Spread your palms, keep your index fingers parallel or slightly turned out, and turn your toes under.

2. Exhale and push your knees up and away from the floor. At first, keep your knees slightly bent and your heels lifted. Lengthen your tailbone away from the back of your pelvis and press it lightly toward your pubis. Against this resistance, lift your sitting bones toward the ceiling, and from your inner ankles draw your inner legs up into your groin.

3. With an exhalation, push your top thighs back and stretch your heels onto or down toward the floor. Straighten your knees, but be sure not to lock them. Firm your outer thighs and roll your upper thighs inward slightly, narrowing the front of your pelvis.

4 Firm your outer arms and press the bases of your fingers actively into the floor. From these two points, lift along your inner arms from your wrists to the tops of your shoulders. Firm your shoulder blades against your back, then widen and draw them toward your tailbone. Keep your head between your upper arms; don't let it hang.

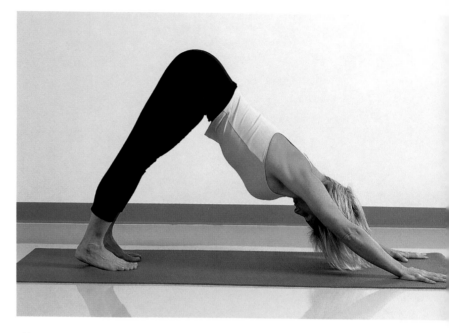

This pose stretches the shoulders, hamstrings, calves, arches, and hands. It strengthens the arms, back, and legs.

Modifications, Variations, and Props

▶ Most beginners struggle to straighten their legs in Downward Facing Dog, but that's not the most important part of the pose. Instead, focus on stretching your back from your butt to your neck in one line, while lifting your butt toward the ceiling. Stretch away from your arms and hands while you lengthen your spine.

▶ To increase the stretch in the backs of your legs, lift slightly up onto the balls of your feet, pulling your heels 1/2 inch or so away from the floor. Then draw your thigh muscles deep into your pelvis, lifting actively from your inner heels. Finally, lengthen your heels back onto the floor, moving your outer heels faster than your inner heels.

▶ To challenge yourself in this pose, inhale and raise your right leg so it's in line with your torso and hold for 30 seconds, keeping your hips level and pressing through your raised heel. Release with an exhalation and repeat on the left for the same length of time.

▶ If you have difficulty releasing and opening your shoulders in this pose, raise your hands off the floor on a pair of blocks or the seat of a metal folding chair.

▶ If you want to do Downward Facing Dog on its own and not as part of the Sun Salutation, stay in it for 1 to 3 minutes. When you're finished, bend your knees to the floor with an exhalation and rest in Child's pose (see page 152).

3

Balancing Postures to Improve Concentration and Memory

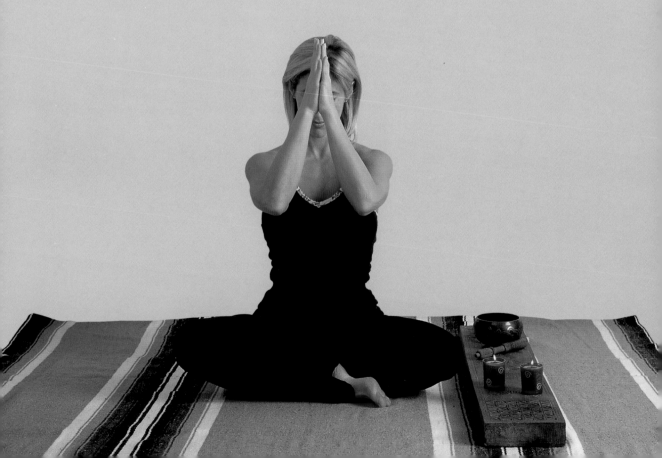

THIS SERIES OF POSES WILL KEEP YOU FOCUSED ON BALANCE IN A NUMBER OF WAYS. YOU'LL BE moving from one side to the other, doing poses standing on your right foot and then your left foot. You'll be moving up and down, balancing on both feet and then on one foot. Moving through these poses will keep your brain challenged.

Early forms of stress-related memory loss have been shown to contribute to the development of Alzheimer's disease. Stress produces a toxic chemical that acts like battery acid on your brain's memory center. The stress-relieving techniques and mind-body exercises of yoga support your body's defenses against stress. Being struck by depression or anxiety, or even just having something traumatic happen, such as a break-up or losing a job, knocks us off balance. We lose our base, be it a job or someone we relied on. Balancing postures teach us that what's important isn't staying straight, but learning how to right ourselves when something seeks to knock us over.

I always tell my students not to worry about losing their balance. You don't have to stay perfectly still and straight during balancing postures. What you have to practice is learning how to let the pose move you a little, but not enough to knock you over. That's balance.

When you're trying to balance, your body and your brain are in deep communication. Your brain is listening to your eyes (Which way is up? Where it the horizon?) and ears (balance has a lot to do with inner ear equilibrium), and even your toes (because it's much easier to balance on one foot when you focus on keeping all five toes on the floor).

Balance work is interesting, too, because thinking about balance won't help you stay straight. In fact, thinking about it will only make it worse. Instead, focus on something outside of you, such as a point on the wall or floor, to keep yourself steady.

And one more thing: When you're not thinking clearly due to anxiety or depression, it's difficult to keep your mind clear enough to remember important dates or tasks. It almost feels as if you're getting dumber (and that's really not going to help you cheer up!) because your brain is so preoccupied with your feelings and your negative thoughts that it's as if there is no room for positive, more important thoughts. Balancing postures will help you regain clarity because your brain appreciates a good workout as much as your body does and, as I said, balancing postures challenge your brain. Also balancing postures, like meditation, give your brain a little vacation by giving it something to focus on besides your feelings, freeing it up to think more creatively. And creative thinking can lead to more hopeful thoughts.

Moving Through

This is a series of poses that flow together just as the Sun Salutation does. Hold each pose for 6 to 10 seconds. Try to move from one pose to the other gracefully and smoothly. You'll move from left side to right side, and then repeat the poses from right to left. This is great for balance and strength.

1. Begin in Mountain, then move into Star by jumping your feet apart and spreading your arms. Be sure to keep your heels placed firmly against the floor and your fingers spread far apart.

2. Return to Mountain and begin to get into Tree by bringing your right leg up.

3. From Tree, extend your right leg into a lunge to get into Proud Warrior.

4. Turn to your right. Turn your right foot out and your left foot in. Tilt over your right leg, right hand just in front of your right foot, left arm up. Look up to your left hand. Lead with your chest and use your strength. This is Triangle, a very powerful pose.

5. Now turn to your left, to balance over your straight left leg in Balancing T. Stretch your arms out behind you. Commit to holding your arms and legs parallel to the floor, which will straighten your back.

6. Turn back to your right side and lunge over your right leg. Bring your arms up over your head and arch your back in Exalted Warrior pose. Tuck your hips under and drop your shoulders.

7. Turn to your left side and go into a forward bend over your left leg. Place your hands in Prayer position behind your back to perform Extended Leg Stretch.

8. Return to the starting position and repeat each pose on the other side.

Star

Like Mountain, Star looks simple—you're merely stretching out your limbs in all directions. But, done properly and with intention, a good Star will not only improve your posture, it will also allow you to breathe more deeply by giving your lungs more room to expand. This is a great stretch to do if you've been sitting for a long time.

1 Begin in Mountain. Open your arms and stretch them out to the sides at the same time that you step your feet out to the sides as wide as possible.

2 Be sure to keep the entire bottom surface of your feet on the floor, being especially careful not to let your ankles roll in. Your pelvis should be tucked under and your hips should be aligned directly under your shoulders.

3 Make sure your shoulders aren't hunched. Beginning from the middle of your back, reach your arms out to both sides. You should feel your upper back spread in two directions, feeling a wonderful stretch in the middle of your back. Your arms should be lifted and you should feel the effort in your triceps.

4 Check that the back of your neck is aligned with your spine and that your head is not tilted forward or back. The front of your body shouldn't collapse in any way. Instead, you should feel it counterbalancing the strength of your spine.

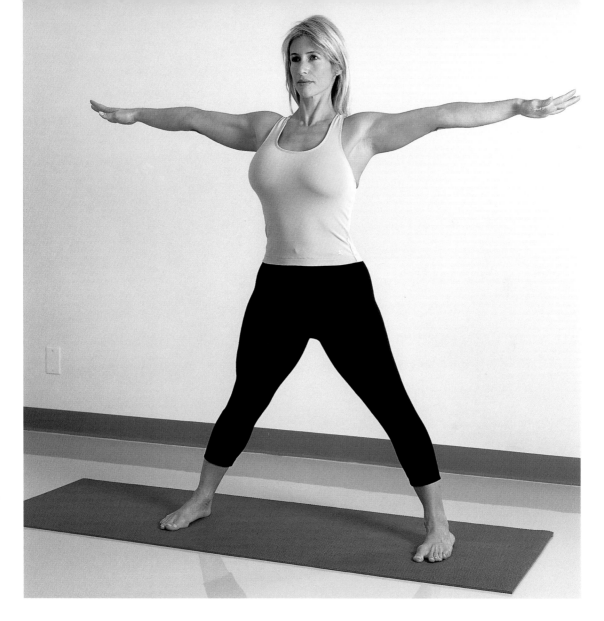

This pose stretches the arm, leg, and abdominal muscles while improving core strength. It also improves posture, strengthens the feet and ankles, tones the buttocks, and releases tension in the spine and neck.

Modifications, Variations, and Props

▶ There is no official modification or prop to use for this pose, but more advanced students can hold it for longer periods of time. A partner can check to make sure you butt isn't swaying out too far behind you and that your pelvis isn't tilted forward.

Tree

One of the most elegant and beautiful of yoga poses, Tree is an invigorating way to practice "being" in a posture. Because it is a balancing posture, many beginning students struggle to stay still and steady. Instead of struggling to achieve this, allow your body to sway a bit, just like a tree in a breeze. This movement will, ironically, help you stay upright. Why? Because attempting to force your body to stay erect only creates stress, and that stress can make you fall. If you give yourself permission to move as necessary, you will be able to work with the natural rhythm of your body to stay tall and relatively still.

1 Stand in Mountain. Shift your weight slightly onto your left foot, keeping your inner foot firm to the floor, and bend your right knee. Reach down with your right hand and clasp your right ankle.

2 Draw your right foot up and place the sole against your left inner thigh. If possible, press your right heel into your inner left groin, toes pointing toward the floor. The center of your pelvis should be directly over your left foot.

3 Make sure your pelvis is in a neutral position, tailbone pointing down, and abdominal muscles contracted.

4 Firmly press the sole of your foot against your inner thigh. Resist with the outer left leg and turn your right knee out as much as possible without turning your hips. Stretch your arms straight up toward the ceiling, parallel to each other and with palms facing. Bring your hands together while keeping your shoulders down and relaxed.

5 Gaze at a fixed point on the floor in front of you, 4 or 5 feet away.

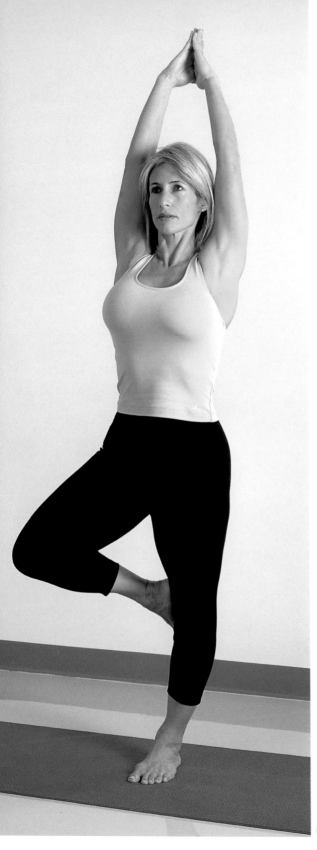

This pose strengthens the thighs, calves, ankles, and spine. It stretches the groin muscles and inner thighs, chest, and shoulders, and it improves balance.

Modifications, Variations, and Props

▶ Don't worry about the placement of your foot in this pose. Different levels of students will place their feet in different places: against the ankle, lower leg, thigh, and even draped across the front of the other thigh are all acceptable positions. Everyone's flexibility and hip rotation is different. The key is to work with your ability as it is now. Over time, your hip and knee will stretch to allow you to change the position as necessary.

▶ You can stand with your back against a wall when you're a beginner doing this pose.

▶ If you're more advanced, challenge your balance by practicing Tree with your eyes closed.

▶ Do not bring your hands up over your head if it is too challenging. Instead, keep them in Prayer (with palms gently touching just in front of your heart) or even on your hips.

Proud Warrior

The challenge in this pose is to keep your legs grounded while reaching out with your arms. Imagine a boxer, who must be steady on his feet and yet free to move quickly and easily. These are the skills all warriors need—even those who only struggle with internal, psychological demons.

1 Stand in Mountain. With an exhalation, step or lightly jump your feet 3 1/2 to 4 feet apart. Raise your arms parallel to the floor and actively reach them out to your sides. Keep your shoulder blades wide and palms down.

2 Turn your right foot in slightly and your left foot out 90 degrees. Align your left and right heels. Firm your thighs and turn your left thigh outward so that the center of your left kneecap is in line with the center of your left ankle.

3 Exhale and bend your left knee over your left ankle so that your shin is perpendicular to the floor. If possible, bring your left thigh parallel to the floor. Anchor your left knee by strengthening your right leg and pressing your outer right heel firmly into the floor.

4 Stretch your arms away from the space between your shoulder blades, parallel to the floor. Don't lean your torso over your left thigh: Keep the sides of your torso equally long and your shoulders directly over your pelvis. Press your tailbone slightly toward your pubis. Turn your head to the left and look out over your fingers.

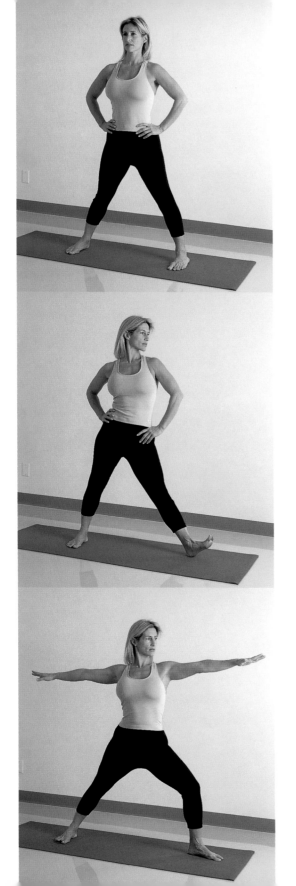

This pose strengthens and stretches the legs and ankles and stretches the groin, chest, lungs, and shoulders. It also stimulates the abdominal organs, increases stamina, and relieves backaches.

Modifications, Variations, and Props

▶ If you have difficulty supporting yourself in this pose, position a metal folding chair outside of your left leg with the front edge of the chair seat facing you. As you bend your left knee to come into the pose, slide the front edge of the seat under your left thigh (taller students may need to build up the height of the seat with a thickly folded blanket). Use the same modification when you perform the pose on your right side.

▶ In the pose described above, your shoulders are centered over your pelvis and the sides of your torso are kept equally long. However, you can also lean your torso slightly away from your left leg, tilting your arms in line with the tops of your shoulders. This stretches the left side of the torso. Use the same modification when you perform the pose on your right side.

▶ When you bend your left knee at a right angle, bend it very quickly and on an exhalation, and aim the inside of your left knee toward the outside of your left foot.

▶ To increase the length and strength of your arms in the pose, turn your palms and inner elbows to face the ceiling while you draw your shoulder blades down your back. Then, maintaining the rotation of your arms, turn your palms from the wrists to face the floor again.

Triangle

This pose is deceptive because it looks easy but it actually challenges you to spread each limb in a different direction while keeping your balance and not leaning forward or back. The goal of the pose is to keep your torso strong and centered. Learning to stay calm in this pose is a good example of how yoga can teach us to deal with life's stresses, because Triangle is almost a physical metaphor for what we must do when confronted by difficult situations. You have to stay in touch with your core, stretch at the same time that you remain strong, and encourage your thinking mind to trust your intuitive mind and body that you can do what's needed and continue doing it for as long as is necessary.

1 Stand in Mountain. On an exhalation, step or softly jump your feet 3 1/2 to 4 feet apart. Land on your heels and make sure the entire bottoms and all toes of both feet rest on the floor before beginning the rest of the pose. Raise your arms out to the sides, parallel to the floor, and extend out from the middle of your torso (so you can feel the stretch in your body) being sure to keep your abdominal muscles contracted and your pelvis tucked under. Keep your shoulder blades down and palms down.

2 Turn your left foot in slightly and turn your right foot out 90 degrees. Keep your legs strong and your hips tucked under. Your body should be in one plane, with no tilting forward or back.

3 Exhale and reach your torso to the right, directly over your right leg. Extend from your hips, rather than bending at the waist. Make sure your hips remain in alignment.

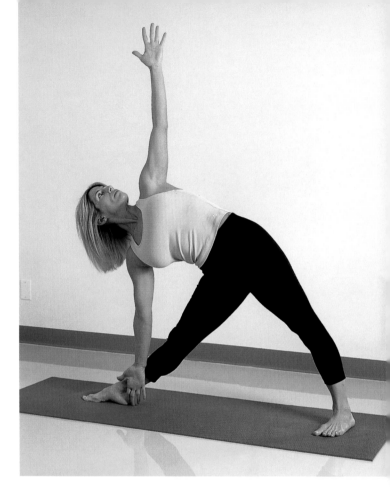

4 Start to tip toward the right and as you bring your right hand to rest on the floor. If you can't reach the floor, rest your hand on your shin or ankle.

5 Stretch your left arm toward the ceiling, keeping your shoulders aligned (so your torso isn't tilting forward or falling back).

6 Turn your head up and look at your fingers or the ceiling without twisting your neck.

7 Inhale to come up, keeping your feet anchored to the floor.

Triangle strengthens the thighs, calves, ankles, and spine while it stretches the groin and inner thighs, chest, and shoulders. It also improves balance.

Modifications, Variations, and Props

▶ Place your back heel or your back against a wall for support if you need it.

▶ If you can't touch the floor when you stretch, use a block to extend your reach to the floor.

▶ To make this pose more challenging, stretch your top arm over your head and ear, parallel to the floor, or align your front heel with the arch of your back foot.

Balancing T

I've included this truly advanced posture because it challenges you to maintain your equilibrium while moving. But don't be intimidated—remember, we all maintain our balance while we walk, dance, run, and play sports. The key to this pose is maintaining a sense of humor and trust. I also believe this is a "brain balancer" because your limbs are going in all directions, including down (against the floor), up (lifting your torso) and forward and back (your torso and arms and legs).

My belief is that if you can keep your body and mind centered in this position, then you will free up your mood to become happier and more balanced—just like the pose itself.

1. Stand in Mountain. Bring your arms up overhead while maintaining your posture. Step your left foot about 2 feet ahead of your body and get centered in this pose.

2. Keeping your abdominal muscles contracted, start to tilt forward while bringing your right leg up behind you. You can keep your standing leg completely straight or slightly bent, whichever is more comfortable for you.

3. Tilt forward as much as you can, aiming to eventually have your torso, arms, and leg in one completely straight line parallel to the floor. Keep your eyes looking toward the floor and your neck in a straight line with your back.

4. To come out of the pose, step back into Mountain, being sure to keep your torso muscles engaged.

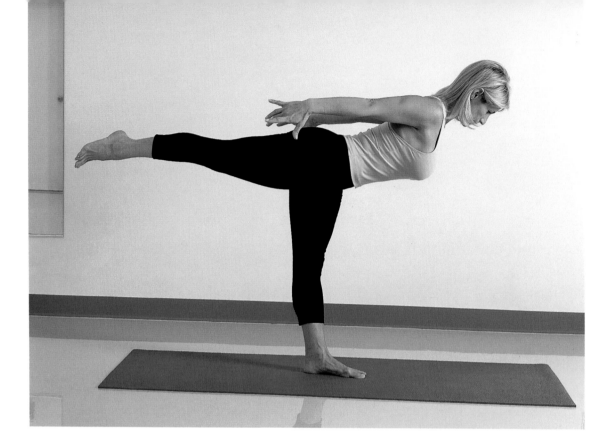

This pose is an excellent stress reliever, as Balancing T requires that the brain release any tension. It's the best leg strengthener of all the standing postures, and it stretches the back and arms.

Modifications, Variations, and Props

▶ People struggle with fear more than anything else in this pose. They believe it is scary, when it is actually easier than it looks. If you need to, practice it while lightly holding onto a chair.

▶ Some people get into the pose best by moving quickly from Mountain to the T position, while others need to move slowly through each position, finding their new center of gravity as they go along.

Exalted Warrior

A more glorious variation of Warrior, in this pose you will focus on stretching your chest as a way of celebrating your strength and future.

1. Stand in Mountain. With an exhalation, step or lightly jump your feet 3 1/2 to 4 feet apart. Raise your arms parallel to the floor and reach them actively out to the sides, shoulder blades wide, palms down.

2. Turn your left foot in slightly and your right foot out by 90 degrees. Align your left heel with your right heel. Firm your thighs and turn your right thigh forward so that the center of your right kneecap is in line with the center of your right ankle.

3. Exhale and bend your right knee over your right ankle, so your shin is perpendicular to the floor. If possible, bring your right thigh parallel to the floor. Anchor your right knee by strengthening your left leg and pressing your outer left heel firmly into the floor.

4. Turn to face over your right leg while bringing your arms together over your head. Gently touch your palms together and stretch back, without crunching your back or neck. Keep the sides of your torso equally long and press your tailbone slightly toward your pubis.

5. Inhale to come back up into Mountain.

This pose strengthens and stretches the legs and ankles; stretches the groin, chest, lungs, and shoulders; and stimulates the abdominal organs. It also increases stamina and relieves backaches.

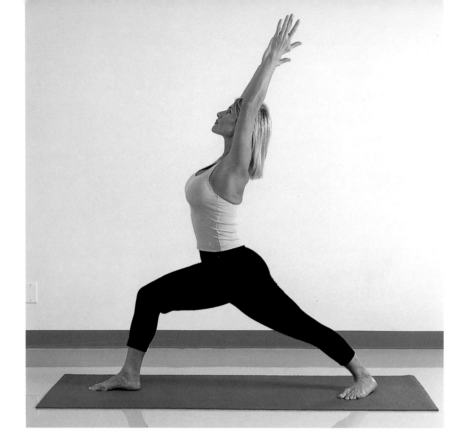

Modifications, Variations, and Props

▶ If you have difficulty supporting yourself in this pose, position a metal folding chair outside of your right leg with the front edge of the chair seat facing you. As you bend your right knee to come into the pose, slide the front edge of the seat under your right thigh (taller students may need to build up the height of the seat with a folded blanket). Use the same modification when you perform the pose on your left side.

▶ Try leaning your torso slightly away from your right leg, tilting your arms in line with the tops of your shoulders. This stretches the right side of your torso. Use the same modification when you perform the pose on your left side.

▶ When you bend your right knee at a right angle, bend it very quickly on an exhalation, and aim the inside of your right knee toward the outside of your left foot.

▶ To increase the length and strength of your arms in the pose, turn your palms and inner elbows to face the ceiling while you draw your shoulder blades down your back. Then, maintaining the rotation of your arms, turn your palms from the wrists to face the floor again.

▶ If it is too challenging to stretch your arms over-head and bend back, focus on keeping your torso upright while keeping your arms at your sides.

Extended Leg Stretch

You would think that it's relaxing, more than anything else, to stretch with intention over one leg. However this pose, like the Warriors on which it is based, requires steady legs and strong abdominal muscles. I suggest letting your mind rest while you focus on maintaining the pull of your legs and abs against gravity—you don't want to sink into the posture.

1. Stand in Mountain. Step your feet wide apart, turning your left foot out and your right foot in, allowing your right heel to sit a little in front of your left heel.

2. Turn your torso toward your left foot, bringing your arms around and placing them in Prayer pose by your lower back.

3. Tuck your pelvis under and contract your abs as you begin to bend from your hips over your left leg.

4. Try to bend down as far as possible, without throwing your back out of alignment with your hips. (In other words, don't sway or arch.) Don't try to force your head down to your knees. Instead, take a few breaths in this position. Each exhalation should allow you to fall forward a little bit more.

5. Slowly return to Mountain.

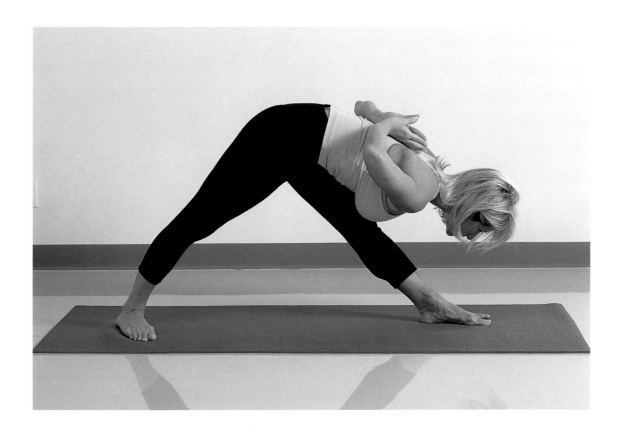

This pose strengthens the legs and relaxes the shoulders, back, and neck. It also tones the abdominal muscles.

Modifications, Variations, and Props

▶ If you can't maintain Prayer position behind your back (if your shoulders are tight it might be difficult), then simply place your hands on your hips.

▶ If you can't keep your back straight or if keeping your leg straight feels painful, you can keep a soft bend in your knees.

▶ If you want to try to come down further but can't keep your hands in Prayer pose, place blocks on either side of your left foot and hold those as you stretch.

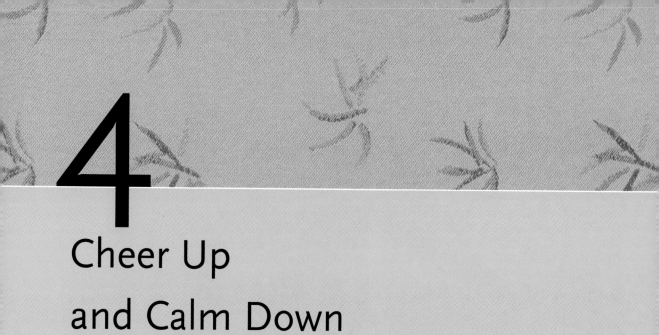

4

Cheer Up
and Calm Down
in 10 Minutes

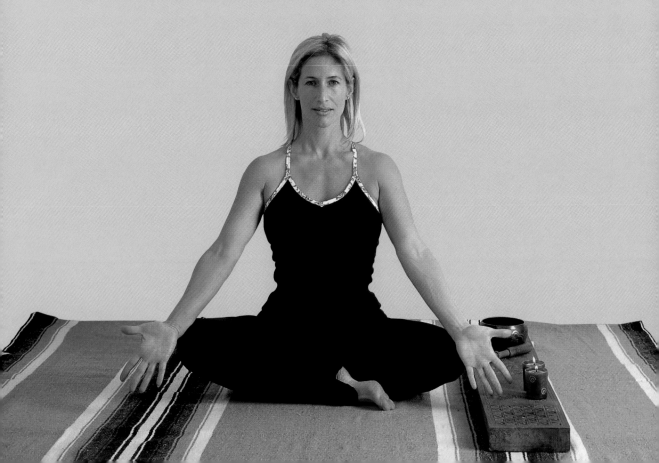

EXCLUDING THE PRESENCE OF A SEVERE DEPRESSION OR THE INTENSITY OF AN ACUTE ANXIETY attack, it doesn't take a long time to change a bad mood to a good mood. And while the effects of a 10-minute workout might not last longer than an hour or so, within that extra 50 minutes of elevated mood you might come up with some more long-term solutions for positive action.

This series of poses will loosen your spine by having you bend and stretch in all directions. Then you'll stretch your legs, and you'll end with a spinal twist that usually gets all the kinks out of your body. And if your body is loose, there's a good chance your mind will be more flexible and happy, too. In other words, you'll be twisted right out of your blues and put into a more positive, happy place.

Moving Through

These postures don't have to link together in a rigid manner. They flow together only inasmuch as they move from gentle stretching to poses requiring more intense flexibility. You should feel free to hold each of these poses for anywhere from 30 seconds to 4 or 5 minutes, depending on your own abilities—they are that relaxing and easy.

Reed

To do Reed properly, you must maintain perfect posture throughout the sequence—even when you're leaning back or bending all the way forward. Proper posture requires you to keep your pelvis tucked under (as if you're squeezing your butt cheeks together very, very slightly) and your abdominal muscles slightly contracted. It should feel as if you have a comfortable girdle holding your torso in. (I say comfortable because you shouldn't feel as if you're clenching anything and you should be able to breathe very deeply.) The final characteristic of good posture is keeping your shoulders down. A lot of people hunch their shoulders toward their ears without realizing they're doing it. In fact, if I were to guess at the most common instruction I give in yoga classes (besides "Breathe"), it would most likely be, "Lower your shoulders."

1 Begin in Mountain with your hands in Prayer pose. Without raising your shoulders, bring your arms up and over your head, palms touching.

2 On an inhalation, pull your shoulders down, tuck your pelvis under, and contract your abdominal muscles as you bend from the waist toward your right. The goal here is to remain in the same plane as your legs and hips, so your torso doesn't twist or bend to the front or back.

3 Hold this pose for a few breaths, then straighten up on an exhalation. Take a breath while standing upright and then bend to the left without tilting forward or back. Be sure your shoulders are lowered, your abdominal muscles are contracted, and your pelvis is tucked under. Inhale as you return to standing straight upright.

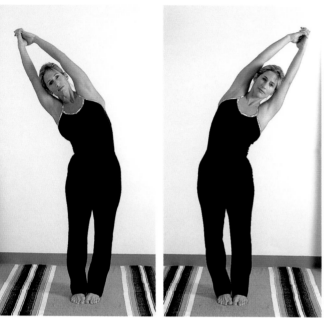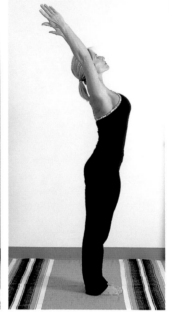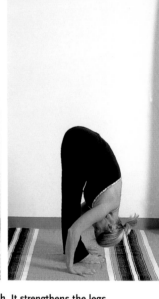

This pose is an all-over muscle stretch. It strengthens the legs and abdominal muscles, as well as the lower-back muscles.

4 Inhale and check that your shoulders are lowered and your abdominal muscles are contracted, then tuck your pelvis under as you tilt backward, leading with the crown of your head and not bending at your neck or waist. Instead of bending, you are reaching with your back. You should strive to keep the line of your body long and elegant. Hold this pose for a few breaths, and on an inhalation, return to standing straight.

5 On an exhalation, reach up and then forward, coming into a forward bend, bending from your hips and reaching your hands to the floor alongside your feet. On an inhalation, return to standing with your arms above your head, and on an exhalation, bring your arms down.

Modifications, Variations, and Props

▶ The best way to do this pose is to have someone watch to make sure that you aren't twisting in your spine or hips. Eventually you will have a "muscle memory" of the way the pose should feel and can do it on your own.

▶ If the back bend is tough on your lower back or neck, check to make sure that you aren't "crunching" your neck or back. Instead, you should be making a long line from your toes to your head, albeit one that has a curve in it (like the Nike swoosh).

▶ If the forward bend is too much for your back, you can hold each bent elbow with the opposite hand as you bend forward (this supports your back) and bend you knees slightly.

Cat and Dog

There is no easier way to get rid of tension in your back than by using Cat and Dog pose. Since you're on your hands and knees rather than holding your body in a standing pose or lying against the floor, your back is free to move forward and back as much as it is able to. It's fabulous!

1 Get on all fours with your shoulders directly over your wrists and your hips directly over your knees. (Don't rely on your own senses to feel this; check your position in a mirror or have someone else check for you.)

2 Keep your pelvis neutral, neck long, and eyes looking toward the floor.

3 Exhale and begin to bring your head and tailbone in toward your belly, arching your back like a cat. Do not bend your neck or hips. Instead, think about creating a long, rounded line along your back from the crown of your head to your tailbone.

4 On your next inhalation, move your back in the opposite direction. Your head and hips should turn up and your back should sway in another long line.

5 Continue moving in this swaying motion with each breath, trying to make your breath cycles last longer and synchronizing the motion of your back with your breath. Repeat as many times as you like, and then come to the neutral starting position.

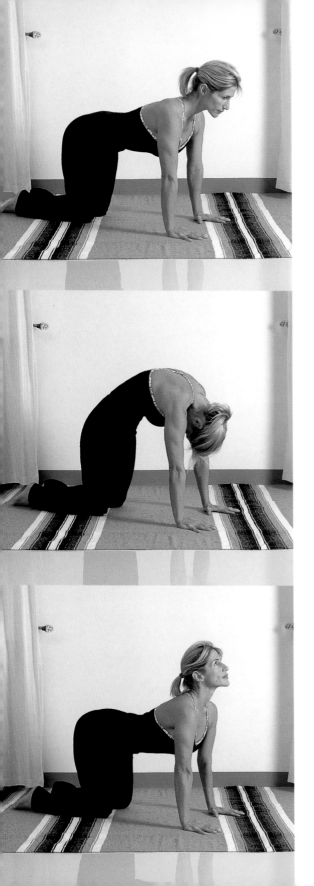

This pose loosens the spine and strengthens the wrists, shoulders, arms, upper back, abdominal muscles, and gluteals. It also releases tension in the back and is great for menstrual cramps.

Modifications, Variations, and Props

▶ Cat and Dog are two of the easiest poses in yoga, so there are relatively few modifications or props necessary. The only people who might be sensitive in this position are those with carpal tunnel syndrome. If you suffer from this, you can do this pose resting on your fists, rather than your palms. (In fact, the fist option works for any pose in which you have to flex your wrists and put weight on your palms.) Yoga has been shown to improve the symptoms of carpal tunnel syndrome, however, you should ask your doctor about specific poses and variations to make sure you are strong enough to do them. Some people who suffer from carpel tunnel syndrome wear wrist pads to protect themselves during their practice.

Open Angle

This is a stretch that everyone, even people who never do yoga, try at one time or another. It looks easy—it's just a spread-eagle pose—but the truth is, it's easy to hurt yourself in this pose because people tend to overextend themselves, imagining that the point of the exercise is to push themselves to the floor. That's not true, however. The point of this exercise is to be calm at the top of the pose and to gradually, over time, with your body leading the way, get to a place where your legs are straight and your back is straight, no matter how much you bend forward. In other words, it's not how far you go, but how you go in the first place that matters.

1 Sit in Staff with your legs extended straight out in front of you, your feet flexed, and your torso perpendicular to the floor.

2 Lean your torso back slightly on your hands and lift and open your legs to form a 90-degree angle. Press your hands against the floor and slide your buttocks forward, widening your legs another 10 to 20 degrees. Rotate your thighs out, pinning your outer thighs against the floor so that your kneecaps point straight up toward the ceiling. Reach out through your toes, pressing though the balls of your feet.

3 With your thighbones pressed heavily into the floor and your kneecaps pointing up toward the ceiling, walk your hands forward between your legs. Keep your arms long. As with all forward bends, the emphasis is on moving from your hip joints and maintaining the length of your front torso. As soon as you find yourself bending from your waist, stop, reestablish the length from pubis to navel, and continue forward if possible.

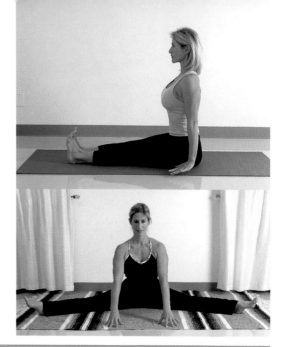

4 Increase the forward bend on each exhalation until you feel a comfortable stretch in the backs of your legs. Stay in the pose for 1 minute or longer. Come up on an inhalation, keeping your front torso long.

This pose stretches the hamstrings, calves, hips, thighs, knees, spine, and groin.

Modifications, Variations, and Props

▶ A beginner might not be able to bring her torso forward toward the floor. In that case, take a bolster or a thickly rolled blanket and lay it on the floor in front of you, its long axis perpendicular to your pelvis. Exhale into the forward bend and lay your torso down on this support.

▶ This pose also has a twisted variation. From the upright position described in Step 1, turn your torso to the right as you exhale. Press your left hand to the outside of your right thigh and your right hand on the floor to the outside of your right hip. With a series of exhalations, walk your left hand down along the outside of your leg. Press the top of your left thigh into the floor to serve as the anchor for this movement. Stop at a comfortable place along the way or, if your flexibility allows it, reach your left hand to the outside of your right foot. Make sure that as you twist to the right and move your hand along your leg you don't shorten your right side. Continue pressing your right hand against the floor to help lengthen that side of your torso. Hold for 1 minute. To come out of this pose,

exhale and pull your torso back to where you started your twist. Then return to upright with an inhalation and repeat to the left.

▶ This is a difficult forward bend for many beginners. If you have trouble bending even a little bit forward, it's acceptable to bend your knees slightly. You might even support your knees on thinly rolled blankets, but remember that it's still important keep your kneecaps pointing toward the ceiling as you move into the forward bend.

▶ Advanced students can help themselves move deeper into the forward bend. Perform Steps 1 and 2 above, then reach out and wrap your index and middle fingers around your big toes, securing each pair of fingers in place with a thumb. Pull back on your toes as you lean forward, but push actively through the bases of your big toes to keep your inner and outer ankles even. Bend your elbows out to the sides and lift them away from the floor as your torso descends.

Lying Spinal Twist

While many of us hold tension in our backs, few of us realize how easy it is to loosen that tension with a twist (and I'm not talking about the kind of twist you put in a martini!). The Lying Spinal Twist always cheers up both my back and my mood because it releases the muscles, as well as the stress I'm storing in them.

1 Lie flat with your lower back gently pressed to the floor. Your shoulders should be attached strongly to the floor and lowered away from your neck.

2 Bend your right knee and bring it up toward your chest, and then tilt toward your left side, keeping both shoulders on the floor. The twist comes from having your upper body remain in place while your lower body twists. (If you let your shoulders come off the floor, you're not really twisting, you're rolling.)

3 Hold the pose for a few breaths, then return to the starting position. Realign your spine and shoulders with the floor before performing the pose to the other side.

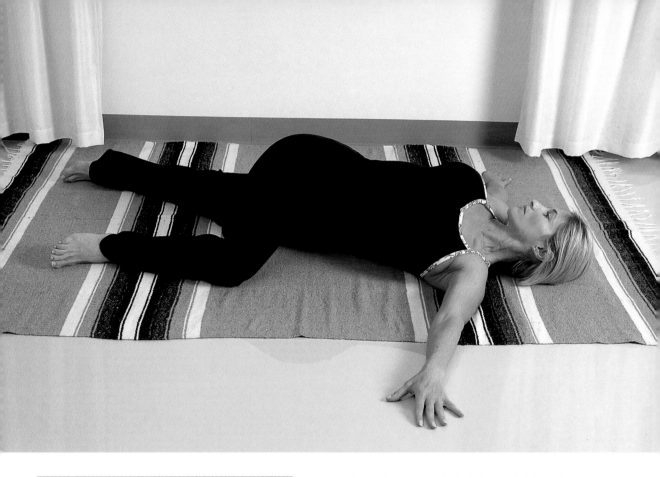

Modifications, Variations, and Props

▶ Few people have trouble with this pose, but if it's tough on your back, you can start with both knees pulled in toward your chest. Then, tilt both knees to one side. They most likely will not go to the floor together, which is fine. The most important objective, with or without this modification, is to keep your shoulders pressed to the floor so that you spine twists.

▶ If it bothers you to let your knees drop together while performing the modification of this pose, you can use one hand as support to hold your knees up.

This pose increases flexibility in back and abdominal muscles, strengthens the core torso muscles, and increases the range of motion in the hips.

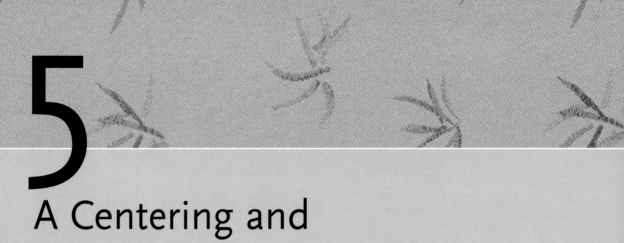

5

A Centering and Challenging 20-Minute Daytime Workout

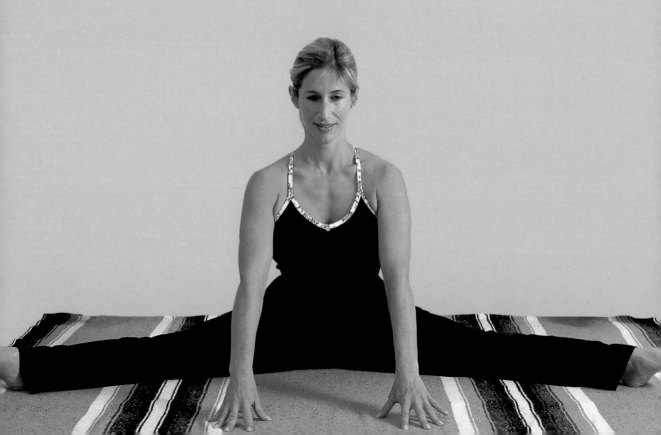

HAVE YOU EVER NOTICED THAT SOME OF YOUR BEST IDEAS COME TO YOU WHEN YOU'RE IN THE middle of doing something else? And it's usually when you're doing something mindless and yet physical, such as taking a shower or walking. A life coach once told me that when one side of your brain is occupied with a repetitive activity, the creative side of your brain is freed up. This exercise routine will keep you moving, and it's tough (certainly tougher than walking and taking a shower), but it doesn't require a whole lot of thinking. So I hope that while you're doing this—especially after you get good at it (and you will)—that it will allow you to let the free place in your mind take over and bring you to a new, happy, hopeful place.

Moving Through

Begin with a few Sun Salutations to warm-up and loosen your spine. (Make sure you do an even number, letting each leg lead the same number of times.) Then move through the remaining poses slowly in the order given here. These poses require some props, but more than that, they require that you surrender to your ability to challenge yourself—you'll be doing inversions (going upside down) as well as holding your body weight up from the floor. But believe me, the rewards—full-body strength and total spinal relaxation—are worth it.

Mountain

Mountain is simply the perfect standing position—whether you're doing yoga or standing in line at the grocery store. Once you begin to stand properly in yoga class, you'll carry this skill into the rest of your life. Good posture is part of the mind-body link: When you stand up properly, your lungs have more room to breathe fully; your spine is supported, taking away small aches and pains; and you feel free to move gracefully.

1 Stand with your big toes touching, heels slightly apart, feet parallel. Rock back and forth and side to side. Gradually reduce this swaying to a standstill, with your weight balanced evenly between your feet.

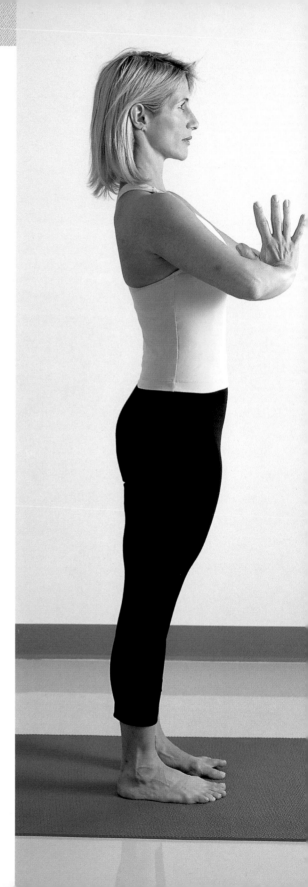

2 Firm your thigh muscles and lift your kneecaps. Bring your hands into prayer position just in front of your chest. Lift your inner ankles to strengthen your inner arches, then imagine a line of energy all the way up along your inner thighs to your groin, and from there through the core of your torso, neck, and head, and out through the crown of your head. Turn your upper thighs slightly inward. Lengthen your tailbone toward the floor and lift your pubis toward your navel.

3 Press your shoulder blades into your back, then widen them across and release them down your back. Without pushing your lower front ribs forward, lift your chest toward the ceiling. Widen your collarbones. Hang your arms beside the torso.

4 Balance the crown of your head directly over the center of your pelvis, with the underside of your chin parallel to the floor, throat soft, and tongue wide and flat on the floor of your mouth. Soften your eyes.

Modifications, Variations, and Props

▶ You can check your alignment in this pose with your back against a wall. Stand with the backs of your heels, sacrum, and shoulder blades (but not the back of your head) touching the wall. Stand straight with your hips tucked under and shoulders down.

▶ You can challenge your balance by practicing this pose with your eyes closed.

▶ You can alter the position of your arms in a variety of ways:

- Hold your hands in Prayer pose, centered in front of your chest,
- Stretch your arms upward, perpendicular to the floor and parallel with each other, with your palms facing inward,
- Interlace your fingers, extend your arms straight out in front of your torso, turn your palms away, and then stretch your arms overhead so your palms face the ceiling,
- Cross your arms behind your back, holding each elbow with the opposite-side hand (be sure to reverse the cross of the forearms and repeat for an equal length of time).

▶ You can improve your balance in this pose by standing with your inner feet anywhere from 3 to 5 inches apart.

Mountain strengthens the entire body, especially the leg, abdominal, and back muscles. It relaxes the shoulder muscles and firms the buttocks.

Standing Forward Bend

New yogis often assume the "point" of this pose is to get your head as close to your legs as possible, but that's not the case. From a physical point of view, your goal in Standing Forward Bend is to maintain good posture, even though you're bent in two. In other words, yoga teachers like to see straight legs (if possible) and flat backs, as well as hips high in the air. From a mental point of view, the point, as in all other postures, is to remain relaxed and breathing deeply throughout the pose.

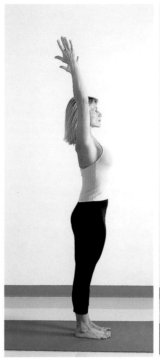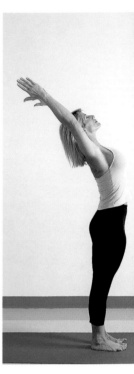

This pose stretches the hamstrings, calves, and hips and strengthens the thighs and knees.

1 Stand in Mountain pose and bring your hands out to your sides and up above your head. Arch your body backward, and then as you exhale, bend forward from your hip joints, not from your waist. As you descend, draw your front torso out of your groin and open the space between your pubis and top sternum. As in all forward bends, the emphasis is on lengthening the front torso as you move more fully into the position.

2 If possible, with your knees straight, bring your palms or fingertips to the floor slightly in front of or beside your feet, or bring your palms to the backs of your ankles. If this isn't possible, cross your forearms and hold your elbows. Press your heels firmly into the floor and lift your sitting bones toward the ceiling. Turn your top thighs slightly inward.

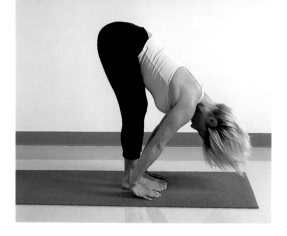

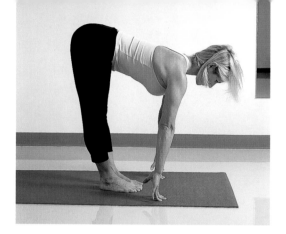

3 With each inhalation in the pose, lift and lengthen your front torso just slightly; with each exhalation release a little more fully into the forward bend. In this way the torso oscillates almost imperceptibly with your breath. As you bend forward, let your head hang from the root of your neck, which is deep in the upper back, between the shoulder blades.

4 After bending forward, slide the index and middle finger of each hand in between the big toe and second toe of each foot. Then curl your fingers under the bottom and around your big toe and wrap your thumb around your fingers. With an inhalation, straighten your arms and lift your front torso away from your thighs, making your back as concave as possible. Hold for a few breaths, then exhale and lengthen down and forward, bending your elbows out to the sides.

Modifications, Variations, and Props

▶ Do this pose with bent knees, or perform it with your hands on a wall, legs perpendicular to your torso, and arms parallel to the floor.

▶ To increase the stretch in the backs of your legs, stand with the balls of your feet elevated an inch or more off the floor on a sand bag or thick book.

▶ If you're performing the pose by itself, don't roll your spine to come up. Instead bring your hands to your hips and stretch your front torso out long. Then press your tailbone down and into your pelvis and come up on an inhalation with a long front torso.

▶ To increase the stretch in the backs of your legs, bend your knees slightly. Imagine that your sacrum is sinking deeper into the back of your pelvis and bring your tailbone closer to your pubis. Against this resistance, push your top thighs back and heels down and straighten your knees again. Be careful not to straighten your knees by locking them back (you can press your hands against the back of each knee to provide some resistance). Instead, let them straighten slowly as you raise your hips.

Bent Knee Lunge/Arms Over the Sun

This is a great all-body stretch that allows you to breathe deeply while you move. This move is also a good warm-up pose for any workout, as it prepares your body for deeper stretches.

1 From the Forward Bend, keep your hands in place on the floor. Step your right foot back as far as possible and bend your left knee, getting into a lunge position. Your left knee should be over your foot, but not past your toes. (You should be able to see your toes if you look down.)

2 Straighten your right leg, keeping the front of your foot and leg down against the floor.

3 Push your hips forward as you release your hands from the floor and bring them up, past the front of your body and over your head. Focus on pressing your right thigh and knee down toward the floor while you're lifting up out of your torso. You should have a real feeling of opposition throughout your entire body: hips pushing forward, legs pressing down, and arms pressing up and back.

4 Be sure to keep your shoulders down and round your spine, as if you're bending back "over the sun," rather than forcing your neck down and toward your back. Your back should make a very rounded C shape as you reach far up with your fingers.

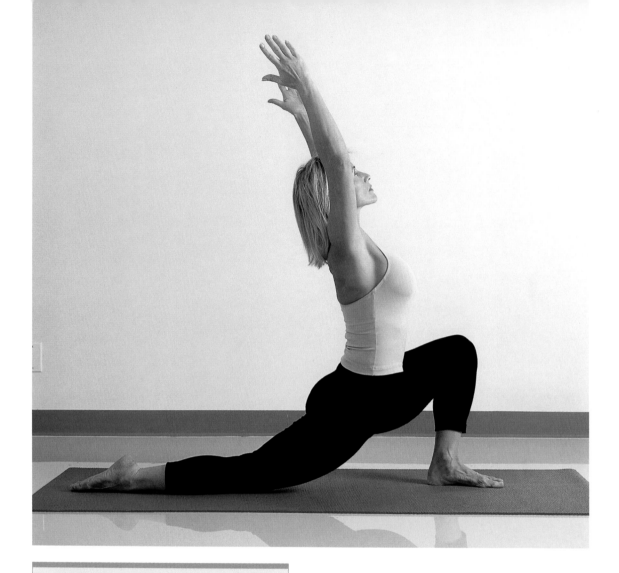

Modifications, Variations, and Props

▶ If you find it difficult to balance in this pose, feel free to keep your hands on the floor or on your bent knee. You can still stretch your spine and shoulders, even though the amount of stretch will be decreased a bit.

▶ You can also keep your straight knee slightly bent, letting just your thigh, knee, and foot touch the floor, rather than the entire leg.

This pose strengthens the back of the body, including the hamstrings, and stretches the front of the body, including the quadriceps, hip flexors, abdominal muscles, pectorals, shoulders, and neck. It increases flexibility and releases tension in the spine. It's a good all-body balancer, as it is done at least twice during any workout, thereby letting each leg stretch and support during a session.

Plank

This is the yoga "push-up." Plank strengthens the entire body, but it is particularly challenging to the core muscles of your torso—the transverse abdominal and back muscles. From a mind-body perspective, Plank asks you to move slowly and with control without sacrificing form.

1 Begin with your hands on the floor, directly under your shoulders. Your toes should be flat on the floor, heels and arches pressed back behind you. Firm your shoulder blades against your back ribs and press your tailbone toward your pubis. Your body should be in a long, diagonal line from your toes to your head. Look down, with the crown of your head facing in front of you and your neck long and relaxed.

2 There's a tendency in this pose to let your lower back sway toward the floor and your tailbone poke up toward the ceiling. Fight this tendency by keeping your tailbone firmly in place and your legs very active and turned slightly inward. Draw your pubis toward your navel. Keep the space between your shoulder blades broad. Don't let your elbows splay out to the sides; hold them close to the sides of your torso and push them back toward your heels. Press the bases of your index fingers firmly into the floor. Lift the top of your sternum and your head to look forward.

3 With an exhalation, bend your elbows and slowly lower your torso and legs to a few inches above and parallel to the floor. Keep your elbows in toward your sides, shoulders pressed down and back, and your neck long.

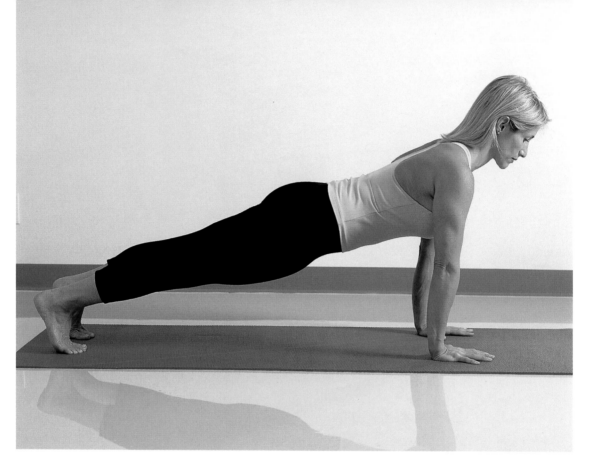

Plank strengthens the arms, wrists, gluteals, and hamstrings. It also tones the abdominal muscles and back.

Modifications, Variations, and Props

▶ You can get a feel for this challenging position by practicing it while facing a wall. Stand a few inches away from the wall and press your hands against it, slightly lower than the level of your shoulders. Imagine that you are trying to push yourself away from the wall, but allow your shoulder blades to prevent the actual movement. Lengthen your tailbone into your heels and lift your sternum toward the ceiling.

▶ Another challenging variation: While performing Plank on the ground, inhale and lift one leg parallel to the floor. Press strongly through your raised heel and lengthen through the crown of your head, keeping your tailbone pressed towards your pubis. Hold for 10 to 30 seconds, exhale your foot to the floor, and then repeat with the other leg for the same length of time.

▶ Open the space between your shoulder blades. As you press your outer arms inward, push your shoulder blades into this resistance. Make sure you don't narrow across the collarbones as you do this.

Cobra

A wonderful stretch for the chest, symbolically bringing joy into your heart, Cobra requires both upper and lower body strength. Its focus on the curve of the back removes a lot of tension from the body.

1 Lie on your belly on the floor. Stretch your legs back, placing the tops of your feet on the floor. Bend your elbows and spread your palms on the floor beside your waist so that your forearms are relatively perpendicular to the floor. Inhale and press your inner hands firmly into the floor and slightly back, as if you were trying to push yourself forward along the floor.

2 On an inhalation, straighten your arms and lift your torso up and off the floor. Keep your thighs firm and turned slightly inward, your arms firm and turned out so your elbow creases face forward.

3 Press your tailbone toward your pubis and lift your pubis toward your navel. Firm but don't harden your buttocks.

4 Lower your shoulder blades and expand chest and sides. Lift through the top of your sternum, but avoid pushing your chest forward. Look straight ahead or tip your head back slightly, but take care not to compress the back of your neck or harden your throat.

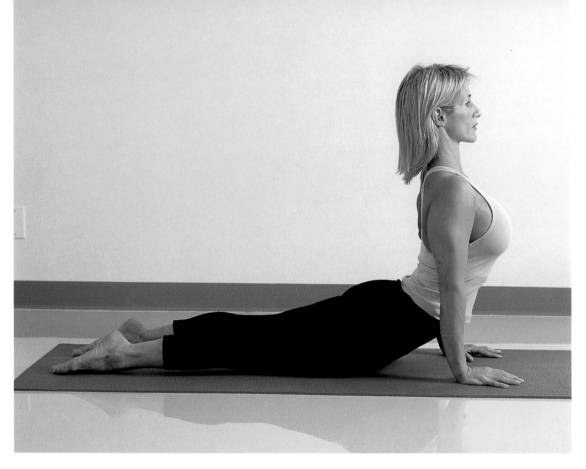

Cobra opens the chest, stretches the shoulders and abdominal muscles, and improves posture. It also strengthens the spine, arms, and wrists, and firms the buttocks.

Modifications, Variations, and Props

▶ You can practice this pose by itself, holding it for anywhere from 15 to 30 seconds while breathing easily. If it's difficult to keep your legs strongly suspended above the floor and you can't remain in the pose for as long as you want to, position a thick blanket roll below your top thighs before you begin the pose. When you are in the pose, lightly rest your thighs on this roll as you press your tailbone closer to the roll.

▶ There's a tendency in this pose to "hang" on your shoulders, which lifts them up toward your ears and crunches your neck. Actively draw your shoulders away from your ears by lengthening down along your sides and pulling your shoulder blades toward your tailbone.

▶ You can also do Upward Facing Dog, a pose similar to Cobra, by pushing off the floor from the tops of your feet and the bottoms of your hands, lifting your legs and lower torso from the floor.

Downward Facing Dog

Possibly everyone's favorite yoga pose, this is the first pose my son learned—as a one-year-old! Downward Facing Dog stretches and strengthens the entire body, releasing tension from every muscle and sore spot. I can't recommend highly enough practicing this pose on its own whenever you feel tense or worried. A partial inversion (part of your body is upside-down), it brings blood to your brain, which can improve your mood while you're working your muscles.

1 Come to your hands and knees on the floor. Place your knees directly below your hips and your hands slightly in front of your shoulders. Spread your palms, keep your index fingers parallel or slightly turned out, and turn your toes under.

2 Exhale and push your knees up and away from the floor. At first, keep your knees slightly bent and your heels lifted. Lengthen your tailbone away from the back of your pelvis and press it lightly toward your pubis. Against this resistance, lift your sitting bones toward the ceiling, and from your inner ankles draw your inner legs up into your groin.

3 With an exhalation, push your top thighs back and stretch your heels onto or down toward the floor. Straighten your knees, but be sure not to lock them. Firm your outer thighs and roll your upper thighs inward slightly, narrowing the front of your pelvis.

4 Firm your outer arms and press the bases of your fingers actively into the floor. From these two points, lift along your inner arms from your wrists to the tops of your shoulders. Firm your shoulder blades against your back, then widen and draw them toward your tailbone. Keep your head between your upper arms; don't let it hang.

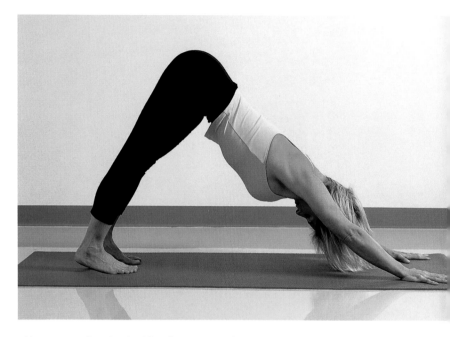

This pose stretches the shoulders, hamstrings, calves, arches, and hands. It strengthens the arms, back, and legs.

Modifications, Variations, and Props

▶ Most beginners struggle to straighten their legs in Downward Facing Dog, but that's not the most important part of the pose. Instead, focus on stretching your back from your butt to your neck in one line, while lifting your butt toward the ceiling. Stretch away from your arms and hands while you lengthen your spine.

▶ To increase the stretch in the backs of your legs, lift slightly up onto the balls of your feet, pulling your heels 1/2 inch or so away from the floor. Then draw your thigh muscles deep into your pelvis, lifting actively from your inner heels. Finally, lengthen your heels back onto the floor, moving your outer heels faster than your inner heels.

▶ To challenge yourself in this pose, inhale and raise your right leg so it's in line with your torso and hold for 30 seconds, keeping your hips level and pressing through your raised heel. Release with an exhalation and repeat on the left for the same length of time.

▶ If you have difficulty releasing and opening your shoulders in this pose, raise your hands off the floor on a pair of blocks or the seat of a metal folding chair.

▶ If you want to do Downward Facing Dog on its own and not as part of the Sun Salutation, stay in it for 1 to 3 minutes. When you're finished, bend your knees to the floor with an exhalation and rest in Child's pose (see page 152).

Bridge

This pose is fabulous for anyone who works at a desk or computer, as it's virtually the opposite of the sitting position. You'll stretch all of the muscles along the front of your body while strengthening the muscles along the back of your body. And there are few exercises—of any style—that are better for lifting your butt. And let's face it, a higher, rounder butt could put a smile on anyone's face, right?

1 Lie on the floor with your knees bent and your feet flat on the floor, heels as close to your sitting bones as possible.

2 Exhale and press your inner feet and arms actively into the floor, pushing your tailbone up toward your pubis, firming (but not hardening) your buttocks, and lifting them off the floor. Keep your thighs and inner feet parallel. Clasp your hands below your pelvis and extend through your arms to help you stay on the tops of your shoulders. Once your shoulders are rolled under, be sure not to pull them forcefully away from your ears, which tends to overstretch the neck. Lift the tops of your shoulders slightly toward your ears and push your inner shoulder blades away from your spine.

3 Lift your buttocks until your thighs are about parallel to the floor. Keep your knees directly over your heels, but push them forward, away from your hips, and lengthen your tailbone toward the backs of your knees.

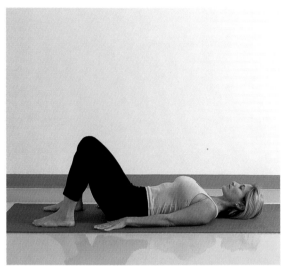 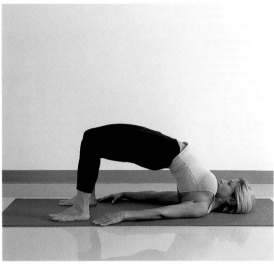

This pose stretches the chest, neck, and spine while it strengthens the back, gluteals, and hamstrings.

4 Lift your chin slightly away from your sternum and, firming your shoulder blades against your back, press the top of your sternum toward your chin. Firm your outer arms, broaden your shoulder blades, and try to lift the space between them at the base of your neck up into your torso.

5 Release with an exhalation, rolling your spine slowly down onto the floor.

Modifications, Variations, and Props

▶ If you have difficulty supporting the lift of your pelvis in this pose, slide a block or bolster under your sacrum and rest your pelvis on this support.

▶ Variation: Once you're in Bridge, exhale and lift your right knee into your torso, then inhale and extend your leg perpendicular to the floor. Hold for 30 seconds, then release your foot to the floor again with an exhalation. Secure your foot again, and repeat with your left leg for the same length of time.

Backbend

Personally, I find few poses as relaxing as Backbend. It could be because I spend so much of time hunched over a computer, as well as holding my son (not that I'm complaining). The backbend opens all of the muscles on the front of your body—it's a more intense version of the previous pose, Bridge. Opening your chest symbolically, and many yogis would say literally, opens your heart to the goodness of the world, which is interesting, because the counterpose (what we do all day when we sit at a desk) covers and compresses your heart. So open up and let in the joy.

1 Lie on the floor with your knees bent and your feet on the floor, heels set as close to your sitting bones as possible. Bend your elbows and spread your palms on the floor beside your head, forearms relatively perpendicular to the floor, fingers pointing toward your shoulders.

2 Press your inner feet actively into the floor as you exhale and push your tailbone up toward your pubis, firming (but not hardening) your buttocks and lifting your buttocks off the floor. Keep your thighs and inner feet parallel. Take 2 or 3 breaths.

3 Firmly press your inner hands into the floor and your shoulder blades against your back and lift up onto the crown of your head. Keep your arms parallel. Take 2 or 3 breaths.

4 Press your feet and hands into the floor, your tailbone and shoulder blades against your back, and with an exhalation, lift your head off the floor and straighten your arms.

5 Turn your upper thighs slightly inward and firm your outer thighs. Lengthen your tailbone toward the backs of your knees, lifting your pubis toward your navel. Turn your upper arms outward but keep your weight on the bases of your index fingers. Spread your shoulder blades across your back and let your head hang, or pull it back slightly to look down at the floor.

6 Stay in the pose for 5 to 10 seconds or more, breathing easily. Repeat 3 to 10 times.

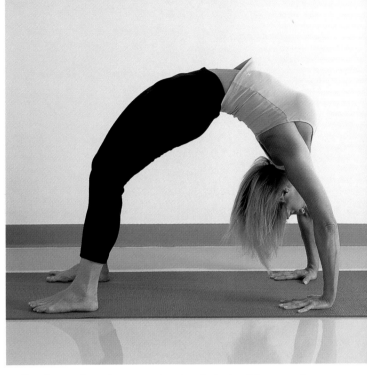

Backbend strengthens the arms, wrists, legs, buttocks, abdomen, and spine while it stretches the chest and lungs.

Modifications, Variations, and Props

▶ Often the armpits or groin are tight and restrict full movement into this pose. In this case, you can support either your hands or feet on a pair of blocks to help yourself realize the full backbend. Be sure to brace the blocks against a wall and if you like, cover them with a sticky mat to keep your hands or feet from slipping.

▶ Once in the pose, lift your heels away from the floor and press your tailbone toward the ceiling. Walk your feet a little closer to your hands. Then press your heels into the floor again to increase the depth of the backbend.

▶ Shift your weight onto your left foot and, with an exhalation, bend your right knee and draw it into your torso. Then inhale and extend your right leg at about a 45-degree angle to the floor. Hold for 5 to 10 seconds, exhale, bend your knee, and return your foot to the floor. Repeat with your left leg for the same length of time.

▶ One variation I love for this pose is to do it on an exercise ball. The ball will support your body, and the arch is perfect for your back.

Supported Shoulderstand

This version of Shoulderstand is performed with a blanket support under the shoulders. It's tough, there's no doubt about it, but it's very relaxing because it reverses gravity's pull on your body.

1 Fold two or more firm blankets into rectangles measuring about 1 x 2 feet, and stack them about 18 inches from a wall. (You can place a sticky mat over the blankets to help your upper arms stay in place while you're in the pose, if you want.) Then lie on the blankets with your shoulders parallel the long edges of the blankets, your head on the floor, and your legs pointed away from the wall.

2 Lay your arms on the floor alongside your torso, then bend your knees and place your feet on the floor with your heels close to your sitting bones. Exhale, press your arms against the floor, and push your feet away from the floor, drawing your thighs into the front of your torso.

3 Continue to lift by curling your pelvis and then the back of your torso away from the floor, so that your knees come toward your face. Stretch your arms out parallel to the edge of the blanket and press your fingers against the floor. Bend your elbows and draw them toward each other. Lay the backs of your upper arms on the blanket and spread your palms against the back of your torso. Raise your pelvis over your shoulders, so that your torso is relatively perpendicular to the floor. Walk your hands toward the floor without letting your elbows slide too much wider than shoulder width.

continued on the next page >

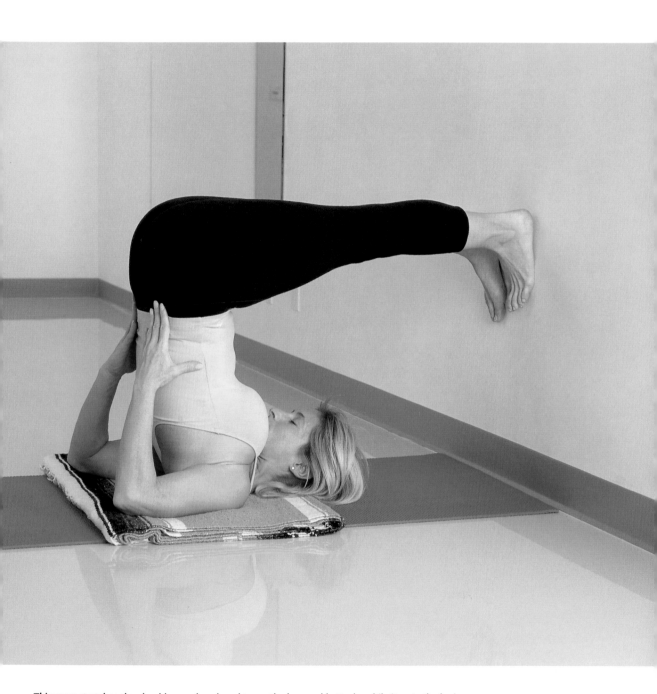

This pose stretches the shoulders and neck and tones the legs and buttocks while it rests the brain.

Supported Shoulderstand *(continued)*

4 Inhale and lift your bent knees toward the ceiling, bringing your thighs in line with your torso and hanging your heels down by your buttocks. Press your tailbone toward your pubis and turn your upper thighs inward slightly. Inhale and straighten your legs, then drop them so the soles of your feet touch the wall and your legs are parallel to the floor. When the backs of your legs are fully extended, lift through the balls of your big toes so your inner legs are slightly longer than your outer legs.

5 Soften your throat and tongue. Firm your shoulder blades against your back, and move your sternum toward your chin. Your forehead should be relatively parallel to the floor, your chin perpendicular. Press the backs of your upper arms and the tops of your shoulders actively into the blanket support, and try to lift your upper spine away from the floor. Gaze softly at your chest.

6 As a beginner, stay in the pose for about 30 seconds. Gradually add 5 to 10 seconds every day or so until you can comfortably hold the pose for 3 minutes. Continue for 3 minutes each day for a week or two, until you feel relatively comfortable in the pose. Again, gradually add 5 to 10 seconds every day or so until you can comfortably hold the pose for 5 minutes.

7 To come out of the pose, exhale, bend your knees into your torso, and roll your back slowly and carefully down to the floor, keeping the back of your head on the floor.

Modifications, Variations, and Props

▶ Rolling up into Shoulderstand from the floor might be difficult at first. You can use a wall to help you learn the pose. Set your blankets up a foot or so from the wall (the exact distance depends on your height; taller students will be farther from the wall, shorter students closer). Sit sideways on your support (with one side toward the wall) and, on an exhalation, swing your shoulders down onto the edge of the blanket and your legs up onto the wall. Bend your knees at right angles, push your feet against the wall, and lift your pelvis off the support.

▶ An easy variation: Come into the pose. Stabilize your left leg perpendicular to the floor, then exhale and lower your right leg parallel to the floor without disturbing the position of the left. The outer hip of your lowered leg (in this case, the right) tends to sink toward the floor. To correct this, turn your right leg outward, moving its sitting bone toward the left. Hold your sitting bones close and rotate your right leg back to neutral from your hip joint. Hold for 10 to 30 seconds, inhale and bring your right leg back to perpendicular, and repeat on your left leg for the same length of time.

▶ Beginners' elbows tend to slide apart and let their upper arms roll inward, which sinks the torso onto the upper back, collapsing the pose and potentially straining the neck. Before coming onto your blanket support, roll up a sticky mat and set it on the support, with its long axis parallel to the edge closest to the wall. Then come up with your elbows lifted on and secured by the sticky mat.

▶ It's common in this pose for students to press only the index-finger sides of their hands against their backs, but be sure you're actually spreading both palms wide against your back torso. Push in and up against your back, especially with your ring and pinky fingers. Periodically take your hands away from your back, press your shoulder blades in, and return your hands to your back a little closer to the floor than they were before.

Seated Forward Bend

This is a pose I strive to perfect—it's a lot harder than it looks and it's particularly tough for people with tight hamstrings and lower backs. But it's precisely those people who should practice this, as it's tough to release tension in those areas. Speaking of tension, don't stress if you can't get as far down as the model does in this pose. Instead, use your breath to gently increase the stretch and you'll find your extension increasing each time you practice.

1 Sit on the floor with your legs straight in front of you, feet flexed. Keep your shoulders down and your abdominal muscles contracted as you extend up through the crown of your head.

2 Inhale. Keep your torso long as you lean forward without bending at your waist, but rather extending over your legs from your hips.

3 If you can, bring your fingers to the sides of your feet, arms extended.

4 When you are ready to go further, don't forcefully pull yourself into the forward bend, whether your hands are on your feet or holding a strap. Always lengthen your front torso into the pose, keeping your head raised. If you are holding your feet, bend your elbows out to the sides and lift them away from the floor. If you're holding a strap, lighten your grip and walk your hands forward, keeping your arms long. Your lower belly should touch your thighs first, then your upper belly, ribs, and finally your head.

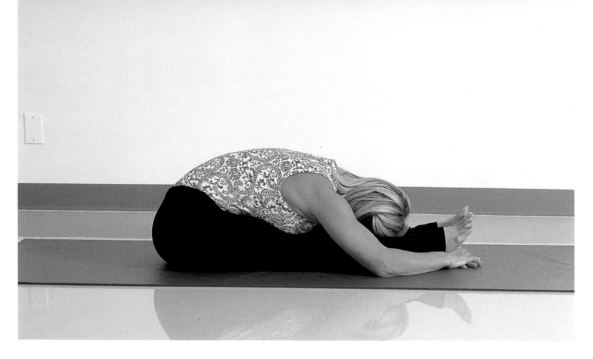

Stretches the spine, shoulders, and hamstrings.

5 With each inhalation, lift and lengthen your front torso just slightly; with each exhalation, release a little more fully into the forward bend. In this way your torso lengthens almost imperceptibly with each breath. Eventually you may be able to stretch your arms out beyond your feet on the floor.

6 Stay in the pose for 1 to 3 minutes. To come up, lift your torso away from your thighs and straighten your elbows again if they are bent. Then inhale and your torso up by pulling your tailbone down and into your pelvis.

Modifications, Variations, and Props

▶ If your legs are not as straight as you'd like and you can't reach completely over your legs (very few people can), try sitting on a folded blanket and holding a strap around your feet to increase the stretch. Don't pull yourself toward your feet, just try to gently breathe through the posture.

▶ If you can get your hands to your feet and want to increase the stretch further still, try to straighten your arms and focus on flattening your back, rather than rounding over your legs.

Headstand

Few poses make me feel as proud as the Headstand. Standing on your head in proper alignment calms the brain and strengthens the body. The key to this pose is to "stand" as straight as you do in Mountain, meaning you'll tuck your tailbone under and gently contract your abdominal muscles. You'll be amazed at how energizing this is to your muscles, which are so used to being held the opposite way, with gravity pulling in one direction for years on end. Headstand is one of the yoga poses I crave—like chocolate.

1 Kneel on the floor. Lace your fingers together and set your forearms on the floor, elbows shoulder-width apart. Roll your upper arms slightly outward, but press your inner wrists firmly into the floor. Set the crown of your head on the floor. If you are just beginning to practice this pose, press the bases of your palms together and snuggle the back of your head against your clasped hands. If you're a more experienced student, you can open your hands and place the back of your head into your open palms.

2 Inhale and lift your knees off the floor. Carefully walk your feet closer to your elbows, heels elevated. Actively lift through the tops of your thighs, forming an inverted V. Firm your shoulder blades against your back and lift them toward your tailbone so the front of your torso stays as long as possible. This should help prevent the weight of your shoulders from collapsing onto your neck and head.

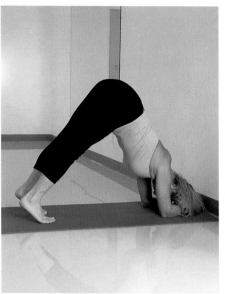 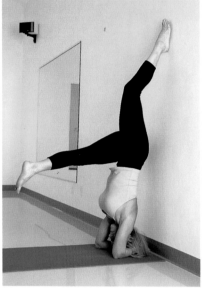 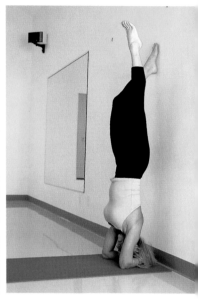

This pose strengthens the arms, legs, and spine, and tones the abdominal organs.

3 Exhale and lift your feet away from the floor. Try to take both feet up at the same time, even if it means bending your knees and hopping lightly off the floor. As your legs (or thighs, if your knees are bent) rise to perpendicular to the floor, firm your tailbone against the back of your pelvis. If you can't lift both legs at once, stabilize one leg against the wall before lifting your other leg. Turn your upper thighs in slightly, and actively press your heels toward the ceiling (straightening your knees if you bent them to come up).

4 Firm your outer arms inward, and soften your fingers. Continue to press your shoulder blades against your back, widen them, and draw them toward your tailbone. Keep your weight evenly balanced on your forearms. It's also essential that your tailbone continue to lift upward toward your heels. Once the backs of your legs are fully lengthened through your heels, maintain that length and lift your right leg away from the wall. Press up through your big toe so your inner leg is slightly longer your outer leg. The center of your right arch should align over the center of your pelvis, which in turn should align over the crown of your head. Hold the pose for 10 seconds.

continued on the next page >

Headstand *(continued)*

5 Bend your right leg and place the sole of your foot back against the wall. Lift your left leg away from the wall, pressing through your big toe and aligning your right arch over your pelvis. Hold the pose for 10 seconds.

6 Add 5 to 10 seconds onto each side every day or so until you can comfortably hold the pose for 3 minutes. Then continue for 3 minutes each day for a week or two, until you feel relatively comfortable in the pose. Again, gradually add 5 to 10 seconds every day or so until you can comfortably hold the pose for 5 minutes.

7 To come out of the pose, exhale without losing the lift of the shoulder blades and touch both of your feet to the floor at the same time.

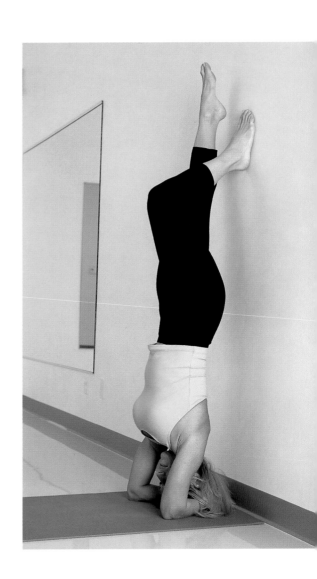

Modifications, Variations, and Props

▶ Balance in this pose is difficult at first, so try to do the pose in the corner of a room, where two perpendicular walls can stabilize your shoulders, hips, and outer heels.

▶ To try a challenging variation, come into the pose and stabilize your left leg perpendicular to the floor. Exhale and lower your right leg parallel to the floor without disturbing the position of your left. The outer hip of your lowered leg tends to sink toward the floor. To correct this, turn your lowered leg outward, moving its sitting bone toward the left. Hold for 10 to 30 seconds, inhale your right leg back to perpendicular, and repeat on your left for the same length of time.

▶ Beginners tend to take too much weight onto the neck and head when coming into and exiting this pose, which is potentially harmful. To come up safely, set your arms in place and lift your head slightly off the floor. Lower your head lightly onto the floor after moving into the wall-supported position. Support 90 to 95 percent of your weight on your shoulders and arms, even if it means staying in the pose for only a few seconds. Over time, slowly take more weight onto your head. When you exit this pose, first lift your head off the floor and then bring your feet down. Eventually you will be able to keep your head on the floor when going up and coming down.

▶ Check the position of your inner wrists. They tend to fall outward in this pose, shifting the weight onto the outer forearms. Turn your pinkies toward the floor, and bring your inner wrists perpendicular to the floor. As you firm your outer upper arms inward, press your wrists actively into the floor.

▶ Have a partner stand to one side and look at the major alignment "landmarks" along the side of your body: your outer ankle bone, the center of your hip, the center of your shoulder, and your ear hole. These points should all be in one line, perpendicular to the floor.

Modified Rabbit Pose

The full version of Rabbit requires you to hold your heels as you "roll" forward, which is pretty tough! In this modified version, you're simply giving your back a fabulous stretch without have to work so hard. Focus as much as possible on breathing deeply through this pose, as people sometimes hold their breath when they bend their neck in this direction. This pose really allows your upper back—a prime spot for tension—to release and expand.

1. Kneel on a padded mat or blanket, keeping your knees and feet together. Point your toes and hold onto your thighs, keeping your shoulders down and your abdominal muscles contracted.

2. Tuck your head down as if you are going to roll forward. Place your palms on your kneecaps and turn your elbows out to the sides.

3. Press your feet and knees into the ground as you "roll" forward, allowing your back and shoulders to spread as wide as possible and forming your body into a C shape. Continue to breathe deeply even though your neck is compressed.

4. Unroll as slowly and easily as possible.

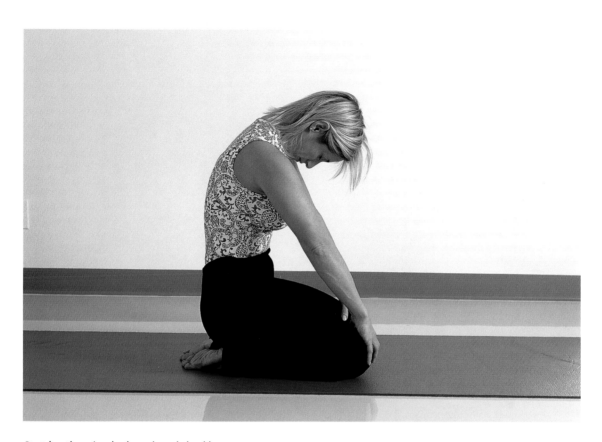

Stretches the spine, back, neck, and shoulders.

Modifications, Variations, and Props

▶ This is the easy version of Rabbit. If you would like to challenge yourself, hold onto your heels, rather than your knees, and bring your forehead to the floor as close to your knees as possible. While you're doing this, lift your butt and hips as high as possible. It's almost as if you are rolling over, but the fact that you're holding your heels stops you. It's very much a feeling of opposition—your head wants to go one way, but your arms are pulling you another—and this is what stretches your back so fully. Your neck will be quite compressed in the front, so try to breathe as deeply as possible and unroll slowly. Do not hunch your shoulders.

Fish

If you hold your tension in your neck, this is the pose for you. It can take a little while to get used to, but it's the perfect release for the neck muscles. I like the way it opens the chest and heart, too.

1 Lie on your back, shoulders and lower back pressed gently toward the floor.

2 Tuck your hands underneath your butt. In one smooth motion, arch your spine and lift your chest while you tilt your head back, reaching the crown of your head toward the ground without crunching your neck.

3 To come out of the pose, lower your shoulders while you slide your head back and lower your chest.

Modifications, Variations, and Props

▶ If your neck and head hurt when you perform this pose, you can put some pillows under your back to mimic the stretch without dropping your neck back.

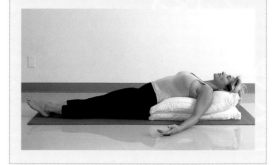

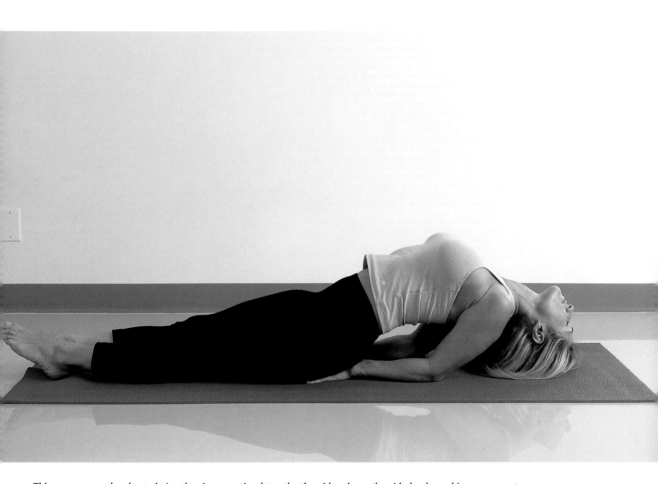

This pose opens the chest, drains the sinuses, stimulates the thyroid and parathyroid glands, and improves posture.

Hero

I've included this gentle sitting posture as a conclusion and a gentle way to decompress after the challenging postures we've just done. But symbolically, it's important to remember that having the courage to face and conquer your blues does make you a hero. My son loves cartoon action movies, and he once asked me why Buzz Lightyear and Woody, the two heroes of the movie *Toy Story*, were heroes. "Because they keep trying," I told him. "They never give up." I think this is the true definition of a hero. One of the great things about yoga is that it's a never-ending practice; no matter where you start, you can always keep going, keep trying. And of course, the same is true with feeling sadness or anxiety. People keep going, knowing that good times and good feelings will come back.

1 Kneel on the floor (on a folded blanket to pad your knees, shins, and feet, if necessary), with your thighs perpendicular to the floor, and touch your inner knees together. Slide your feet slightly wider apart than your hips, with the tops of your feet flat on the floor. Angle your big toes slightly in toward each other and press the top of each foot evenly into the floor.

2 Exhale and sit back halfway, with your torso leaning slightly forward. Wedge your thumbs into the backs of your knees and draw the flesh of your calf muscles toward your heels. Then sit down between your feet.

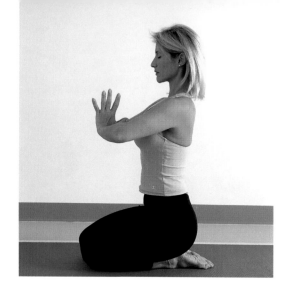

This pose stretches the thighs, knees, and ankles. It also strengthens the arches.

3 If your butt doesn't comfortably rest on the floor, support yourself on a block or thick book placed between your feet. Make sure both sitting bones are evenly supported. Don't rest on your legs; try to keep your hips and thighs energized over your calves by sitting up with your torso while gently pressing your lower legs into the mat. Place your hands in Prayer pose over your heart center.

4 Firm your shoulder blades against your back ribs and lift the top of your sternum like a proud warrior. Widen your collarbones and release your shoulder blades away from your ears.

5 Begin by staying in this pose for 30 seconds to 1 minute. Gradually extend your stay up to 5 minutes.

6 To come out of the pose, press your hands against the floor and lift your buttocks up slightly above your heels. Cross your ankles underneath your buttocks, sit back over your feet and onto the floor, and stretch your legs out in front of you. It may feel good to bounce your knees up and down a few times on the floor.

Modifications, Variations, and Props

▶ If your ankles hurt in this pose, roll up a towel and place it underneath them before you sit back. Clasp your hands, extend your arms forward (perpendicular to your torso and parallel to the floor), turn your palms away from your torso (so your thumbs point to the floor), and on an inhalation raise your arms perpendicular to the floor, palms facing the ceiling. Stretch actively through the bases of your index fingers.

▶ Often the inner top feet press more heavily into the floor than the outer top feet. Press the bases of your palms along the outer edges of your feet and gently push them to the floor to correct this.

▶ Cup your hands around your knees, straighten your arms fully, and pull on your knees. Firm your shoulder blades against your back, lift the top of your sternum, and release your chin down onto your chest without straining the back of your neck. Hold for 10 to 20 seconds. Then let go of your knees and raise your head back to neutral without losing the lift of the sternum.

6

A Relaxing Evening Routine

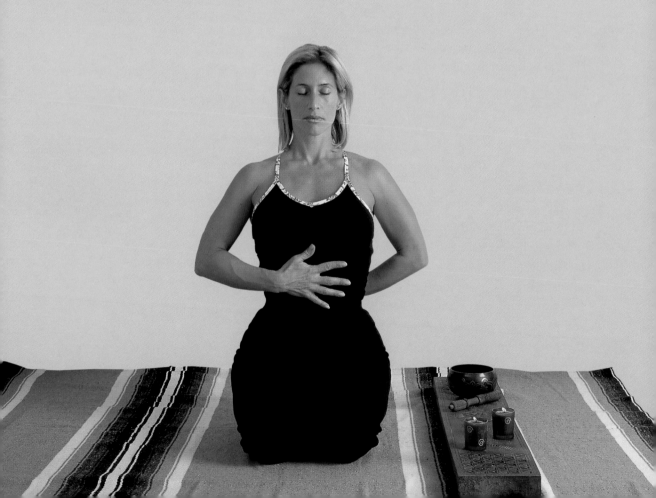

I GREW UP IN A HOME WHERE THE TV WAS ON IN MOST OF THE ROOMS BEFORE WE WENT TO sleep and while we slept. I was different—I fell asleep to the radio—and I never got a good night's sleep. In my early 20s, I decided that I was tired of not being able to sleep—pun intended—and I began to train myself to sleep well. These days, I rarely suffer from insomnia. In fact, I not only have restful nights, but I actually look forward to sleeping because most of my dreams are peaceful, too.

For me, the keys to a good night's rest are in my room's design (a big bed with lots of covers and no TV) and the way I spend my evening hours. I like to exercise a bit in the evening, but I don't do anything strenuous—in fact, yoga is my evening routine, and I don't eat after 6 p.m. (I go to bed early, though. Most sleep experts recommend not eating for two to three hours before you retire, so you'll want to adjust that time accordingly.)

This yoga routine is very gentle and relaxing. It's not designed to improve your physique or tone your muscles. Instead, it will lower your heart rate and, I hope, calm your mind.

Poor, fitful sleep is a hallmark of depression and anxiety. If you find it difficult to get a good night's sleep, do not turn to sleeping pills for anything more than a few days—they can make you groggy, and they won't solve the problem. Instead, try to develop habits that promote good sleep—sleep in a quiet, dark, and cool (but not cold) room, and avoid alcohol before bedtime. (It will help you fall asleep, but won't help you stay asleep.)

Moving Through

These poses don't need to be done in a flowing sequence, although they are all performed on the floor. You can also do them on your bed—in fact, try doing them in the middle of the night if you wake up and can't get back to sleep.

Reclined Bound Angle

This, to me, is the most relaxing pose in yoga today because it specifically opens the two areas of the body that most of us, in today's world, keep contracted and closed: the hips and the chest. We shorten our hip flexors when we sit (at a computer or in the car) and we hunch over that same computer and our steering wheels, which compresses our chest. This is a pose I practice every night, sometimes with the pillow on my bed, just to expand my heart.

1 Fold a firm blanket several times and place it on the floor. Lie on your back in a comfortable position with the blanket under your torso. Inhale and exhale slowly and regularly, making a conscious effort to make your breaths longer and deeper as you practice the pose.

2 With your hands, grip the tops of your thighs and rotate your inner thighs out and away from the sides of your torso. Next slide your hands along your outer thighs toward your knees, and widen your knees away from your hips. Imagine that your inner groin muscles are sinking into your pelvis. Push the front of your hips together, so that the back of your pelvis widens while the front of your pelvis narrows. Lay your arms on the floor, palms up, at about a 45-degree angle from the your torso.

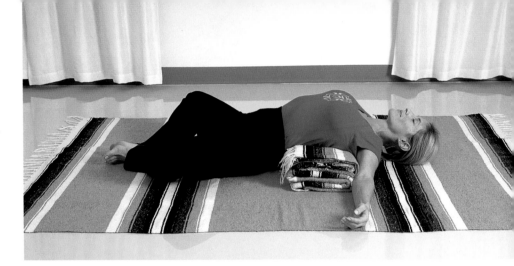

This pose stimulates the organs in the torso and improves general circulation. It also stretches the inner thighs, groin, and knees while relaxing the brain and muscles.

3 The natural tendency in this pose is to push your knees toward the floor in the belief that this will increase the stretch of the inner thighs and groin. But if your groin muscles are tight, pushing the knees down will have the opposite effect: The groin muscles will harden, as will your belly and lower back. Instead of pushing down, imagine that your knees are floating up toward the ceiling and continue settling your groin deep into your pelvis. As your groin drops toward the floor, so will your knees.

4 To start, stay in this pose for 1 minute. Gradually extend the length of the pose to 5 to 10 minutes.

5 To come out of the pose, use your hands to press your thighs together, then roll to one side and push yourself away from the floor, your head trailing your torso.

Modifications, Variations, and Props

▶ If you feel any strain in your inner thighs, support each of your thighs on a block or folded blanket. Make sure the supports, whether blocks or blankets, are the same height.

▶ Support your head and neck on a blanket roll or bolster, if needed.

▶ If it's more comfortable, bring your heels to the floor and press through your feet to lift your pelvis slightly up. Position a block under your pelvis, lower your sacrum onto the block, and drop your knees out to the sides again, pressing the soles of your feet back together.

▶ To be sure that your back is in proper alignment, inhale and raise your arms toward the ceiling, parallel to each other and perpendicular to the floor. As your raise your arms, your shoulders should spread against the floor, widening. Lower your arms back down without losing the space between your shoulder blades.

Leg Squeezes

I love to introduce this pose to my yoga students because its true name, or at least its more poetic name, is Wind Relieving Pose. In other words, if you've got a bit of gas to get rid of, get right into your Leg Squeezes—you'll feel better in no time (and, in fact, pushing a baby's legs gently into these poses will help her get rid of gas in her tummy, too).

But, of course, that's not why I'm including this pose in this book. Well, not exactly. I'm including it because many of us carry tension in our lower backs, and this pose stretches your lower back. Also, when we're anxious, we often get upset stomachs, and as I mentioned, these poses will help ease any problems in your belly.

Mostly, however, I'm recommending these poses because they are a gentle opportunity to rest and relax. So don't worry about getting a good stretch during your Leg Squeezes. Instead, try to imagine the White Light Meditation (see page 36) while you do them and let your inner light bring some rest to you before you sleep.

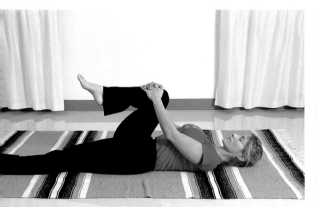 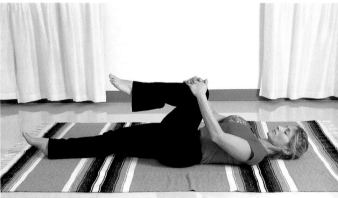

Leg Squeezes stretch the lower back and hamstrings. They also tone the abdominal muscles, relax the shoulder and chest muscles, align the spine, and ease tension in the neck.

1. Lie on your back and bend your knees in order to press your lower back gently to the floor.

2. Straighten your legs as much as possible without (this is very important) allowing your lower back to come up off the floor too much. (It will a little bit, but you should be sure that you don't feel any part of your back tilting.) Let the floor support you. Try to let your muscles ease into the floor as much as possible.

3. On an inhalation, bring your right knee in toward your chest, holding your leg below your knee with both hands. Keep your left leg as straight as possible, but not tense. Hold your right leg gently, and, if you want, move it around to release the tension in your hips and torso.

4. Slowly release your right leg to the floor and bring your left leg in toward your torso. After you've held it in toward your chest for a few moments (or up to a few minutes, if you like), release your left leg.

continued on the next page >

Leg Squeezes *(continued)*

5 Now, bring your right leg back to your chest, but try to straighten your leg, holding it wherever you are comfortable. Try not to hold your leg at a joint (knee or ankle). Once again, be sure your lower back is pressed gently toward the floor. Feel free to pull your leg in toward your chest as you continue to breathe, to increase the stretch.

6 Release your right leg and bring your left leg into the straight-leg stretch.

7 Now, bring your right leg back up, and hold your toes or the outer edge of your foot with the fingers of your right hand. Without turning your back or tilting your hips, let your right leg drop gently to the right side to stretch your right inner thigh and groin. Keep your back pressed gently to the floor, and place your left hand on your left hip to keep if from coming off the ground, if necessary. Return to the start position.

8 Bring your left leg up and repeat on that side. Hold for a few breaths, keeping your back against the floor. Return to the start position.

9 Now, bring both legs to your chest, being sure your lower back is pressed gently to the floor.

10 Extend your legs up straight and then lower them down slowly.

Modifications, Variations, and Props

▶ It is very important that you not sacrifice the line of your back because you're worried about keeping your legs completely straight during this pose. Most people need to have their knees bent in order to keep their lower back pressed into the floor, so be sure to modify your position as necessary.

▶ Do not worry about where you can reach to hold your leg. Remember, your intention during these poses is to relax, not to judge yourself. You will get "results," meaning that your lower back and legs will stretch no matter how far you go, but you will only relax if you let go of your idea of what the pose "should" look like.

▶ If you can't keep your lower back pressed gently into the floor, lie on a blanket to support your back.

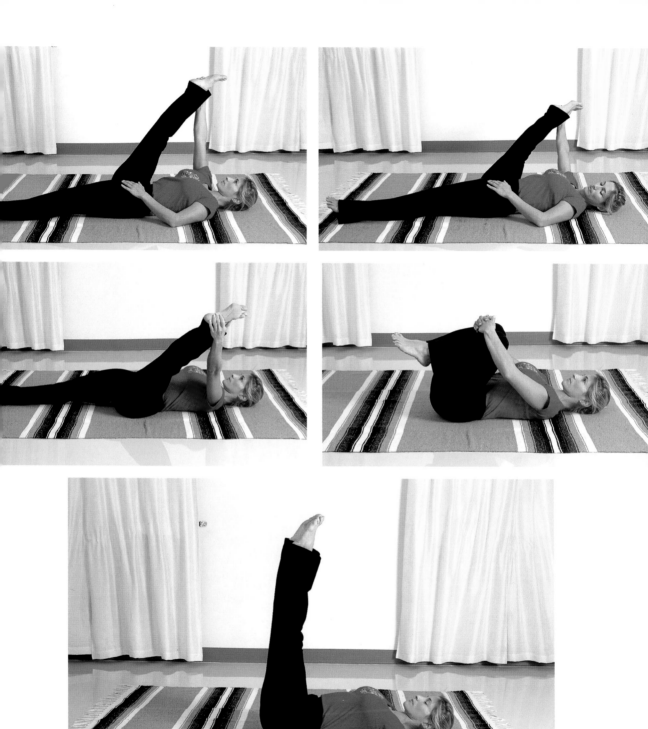

Rest

More commonly called Corpse, this is a pose of total relaxation. Unfortunately, you would be surprised at how many people end up feeling anxious about relaxing! But if you do it properly, you won't want to ever come out of this pose.

1 In Rest, it's essential that your body be in a neutral position. Sit on the floor with your knees bent and feet on the floor, and lean back onto your forearms. Lift your pelvis slightly off the floor and, with your hands, push the back of your pelvis toward your tailbone and then return your pelvis to the floor. Inhale and slowly extend your right leg, then your left, pushing through your heels. Release both legs, softening your groin muscles, and see that your legs are angled evenly away from the midline of your torso and that your feet turn out evenly. Soften (but don't flatten) your lower back.

2 With your hands, lift the base of your skull away from the back of you neck and release the back of your neck down toward your tailbone. If you have any difficulty doing this, support the back of your head and neck on a folded blanket. Broaden the base of your skull, too, and make sure your ears are equidistant from your shoulders.

3 Reach your arms toward the ceiling, perpendicular to the floor. Rock slightly from side to side and broaden your back ribs and shoulder blades away from your spine. Then release your arms to the floor, angled evenly away from your torso. Turn your arms outward and stretch them away from the space between your shoulder blades. Rest the backs of your hands on the floor. Make sure your shoulder blades are resting evenly on the floor, and spread your collarbones.

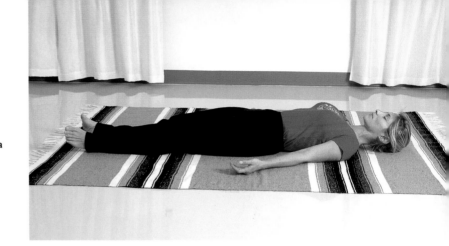

Like its name implies, Rest relaxes the body, calms the brain, and helps relieve stress and even mild depression. It also reduces headache, fatigue, and insomnia and helps to lower blood pressure.

4 In addition to quieting your physical body in Rest, it's also necessary to pacify your sense organs. Soften the root of your tongue, the wings of your nose, the channels of your inner ears, and the skin of your forehead, especially around the bridge of your nose and between your eyebrows. Let your eyes sink to the back of your head, then turn them downward to gaze at your heart. Release your brain to the back of your head.

5 Stay in this pose for 5 minutes for every 30 minutes of practice you've done. Rest should conclude both your asana and your pranayama practices.

6 To come out of the pose, exhale and roll gently onto your right side. Take 2 or 3 breaths. With another exhalation, press your hands against the floor and lift your torso, trailing with your head. (Your head should always come up last.

Modifications, Variations, and Props

▶ If you have trouble relaxing in this pose, it might help to do a progressive relaxation, where you systematically move through all the parts of your body, relaxing them one at a time.

▶ Rest is usually performed with the legs turned out, though sometimes after a practice session involving lots of outward rotation of the legs (as for standing poses), it feels good to do this pose with the legs turned in. To do this, take a strap and make a small loop in one end of it. Sit on the floor with your knees slightly bent and slip the loop over your big toes. Lie back and turn your thighs inward, sliding your heels apart. The loop will help maintain the inward turn of your legs.

▶ Often it's difficult to release the thighs and soften the groin in this pose. This difficulty creates tension throughout the body and restricts the breath. Take two 10-pound sand bags and lay one across the top of each thigh, parallel to the crease of the groin. Then imagine that the heads of your thighbones are sinking away from the weight, down into the floor.

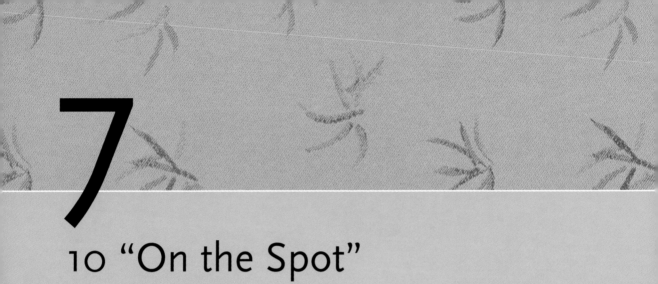

7

10 "On the Spot" Solutions

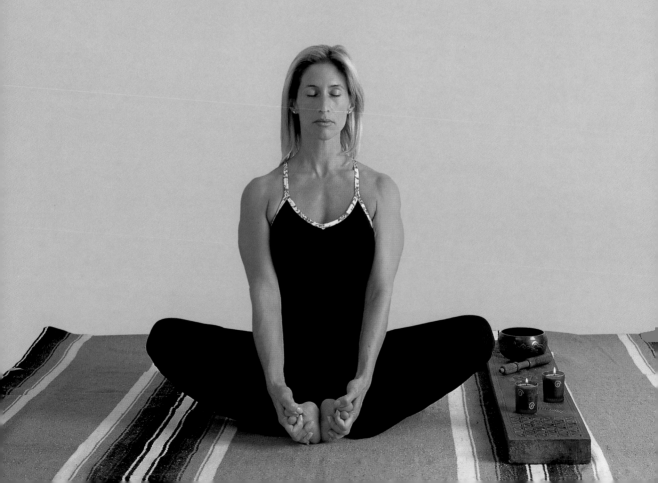

I DESIGNED THESE 10 POSTURES AND POSTURE SEQUENCES TO PROVIDE IMMEDIATE RELIEF IN specific situations. Although each of those poses are done in yoga classes and can be done as part of a series, I am using them differently here. Because many people suffering from depression and anxiety have specific moments in which their symptoms appear, I thought it was important to offer these poses as solutions to specific problems, such as feeling nervous in a crowded room or trying to work through a cloud of sadness.

TO ENERGIZE

Chair With Exalted Arms

Chair looks easy—all you're doing is "sitting." But without a real chair underneath you, your legs have to work to hold your body steady. Raising your arms above your head takes this grounding pose and brings it into the sky.

1 Stand in Mountain. Inhale and raise your arms above your head, perpendicular to the floor. Either keep your arms parallel, palms facing inward, or bring your palms together.

2 Exhale and bend your knees, trying to make your thighs as parallel to the floor as possible. Your knees will project out over your feet and your torso will lean slightly forward over your thighs, forming approximately a right angle with the tops of your thighs. Keep your inner thighs parallel to each other and press down through your heels.

3 Firm your shoulder blades against your back. Take your tailbone down toward the floor and in toward your pubis to keep your lower back long.

4 Hold this pose for 30 seconds to 1 minute.

5 To come out of the pose, inhale and straighten your knees, lifting strongly through your arms. Exhale and release your arms to your sides into Mountain.

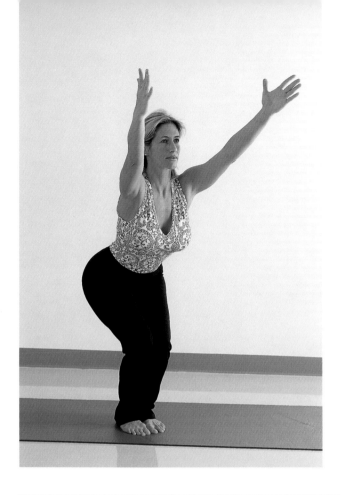

This pose strengthens the ankles, thighs, calves, and spine while it stretches the shoulders and chest. It also stimulates the abdominal organs, diaphragm, and heart.

Modifications, Variations, and Props

▶ You can build strength in your thighs by squeezing a block or thick book between them during this pose.

▶ For a challenging variation, as you bend your knees, come up onto the balls of your feet and sit your buttocks down on your raised heels. Extend your arms forward, parallel to each other and the floor, palms down or facing toward each other.

▶ As a beginner, you may have better luck staying in this pose if you perform it near a wall. Stand with your back a few inches away from the wall, adjusting your position so that when you bend into the pose, your tailbone just touches and is supported by the wall.

▶ To get comfortable in Chair, bring your hands to your thighs. Nestle the bases of your palms into the creases at the tops of your legs, and push the tops of your thighs toward your heels, digging your heels deep into the floor. (A partner can use either hands or feet to press your heels firmly into the ground.) Against these actions, lift your sitting bones up into your pelvis by performing a slight pelvic tilt.

TO OPEN YOUR HEART

Camel

I think Camel is immediate proof that yoga—the system of bodily exercises, not just the meditation and breathing—can change the way you feel inside. Camel opens your chest and, by extension, allows your heart to expand. Somehow, after Camel pose you feel more hopeful and open to life's positive and hopeful possibilities.

1 Kneel on the floor with your knees hip-width apart and your thighs perpendicular to the floor. Rotate your thighs inward slightly and firm but don't harden your buttocks. Imagine that you're drawing your sitting bones up into your torso. Keep your outer hips as soft as possible as you press your shins and the tops of your feet firmly into floor.

2 Rest your hands on the back of your pelvis, bases of your palms on the top of your buttocks, fingers pointing down. Use your hands to spread the back of your pelvis and lengthen it down through your tailbone. Then lightly push your tail forward, toward your pubis. Make sure though that your groin doesn't "puff" forward. To prevent this, press your front thighs back, countering the forward action of your back. Inhale and lift your chest by pressing your shoulder blades against your back ribs.

3 Now lean back against the firmness of your tailbone and shoulder blades. For the time being, keep your head up, chin near your sternum, and hands on your pelvis. Touch your hands to your feet as you keep your thighs perpendicular to the floor. If you need to, tilt your thighs back a little from perpendicular and minimally twist to one side to get one hand on the same-side foot. Then press your thighs back to perpendicular, turn your torso back to neutral, and touch the second hand to its foot. If you're not able to touch your feet without compressing your lower back, turn your toes under and elevate your heels.

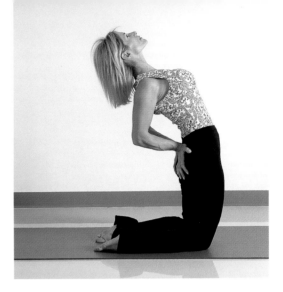

This pose stretches the entire front of the body, ankles, thighs and groin, abdomen and chest, throat, and deep hip flexors. It also strengthens the back muscles, improves posture, and stimulates the organs of the abdomen and neck.

4 See that your lower front ribs aren't protruding sharply toward the ceiling, which hardens the belly and compresses the lower back. Release your front ribs and lift the front of your pelvis up toward your ribs. Then lift your lower back ribs away from your pelvis to keep the lower spine as long as possible. Press your palms firmly against your soles or heels, with the bases of your palms on your heels and your fingers pointing toward your toes. Without squeezing your shoulder blades together, turn your arms out so your elbow creases face forward. You can keep your neck in a relatively neutral position, neither flexed nor extended, or you can drop your head back. Just be careful not to strain your neck and harden your throat.

5 Stay in this pose for anywhere from 30 seconds to 1 minute.

6 To come out of the pose, bring your hands to the front of your pelvis. Inhale and lift your head and torso up by pushing your hip points down toward the floor. If your head is back, lead with your heart to come up, not by jutting your chin toward the ceiling and leading with your brain. Rest in Child's Pose for a few breaths. (See page 152.)

Modifications, Variations, and Props

▶ Camel can be tough for beginners, as they often struggle to reach their heels with their hands, as well as to push their hips forward and stretch their shoulders. The easiest variation is probably more common than the final posture I've shown here. Simply keep your hands on your lower back and push your hips gently forward, dropping your neck back and keeping your shoulders lowered (not hunched around your ears). The most important part of this pose is to stretch your quadriceps and hip flexors (the fronts of your thighs and hips) rather than worry about dropping your head and neck back. The arch in your back will come naturally once you focus on your legs.

TO CALM DOWN

Locust Series

Although you are on your belly for this pose, you are actually doing a backbend. This is a wonderful way to strengthen your back because it's simultaneously strengthening and relaxing. A lot of beginners think the "point" of the pose is to lift their arms and legs as high as possible, but that's not true. The point is to let your breath do the work, rather than your body. You should use your inhalations to lift your arms and legs, and then, while they are still aloft, allow them to drift down as you exhale, naturally rising up again as you inhale. Once you master this in Locust, you will be able to see and feel the power of your breath in other poses.

1 Lie face down on the floor, with your arms alongside your body, palms and forehead down. Bring your knees and ankles together. Squeeze your shoulder blades together and down. Push your palms into the floor. Pull your abdominal muscles inward, contract your buttocks, and press your hips and pubis firmly into the floor. On your next inhalation, raise your left arm and right leg to a comfortable height.

2 As you breathe, allow your limbs to move with your breath. In other words, don't hold your breath or try to hold your limbs still and in one position. Instead, focus on breathing deeply, rather than holding your arm and leg still.

3 Exhale as you slowly lower your arm and leg. Take another full breath and on your next inhalation, raise your right arm and left leg. Exhale and lower them slowly.

This pose strengthens the entire back, increases flexibility in the spine, and stretches the abdominal, chest, shoulder, and quadricep muscles.

4 Lower your face to the floor. Take another full breath and raise your legs away from the floor, keeping your face lowered. Once again, let your breath lead your body.

5 Extend the front of your body as you pull your shoulder blades together, raising your head, arms, and upper torso away from the floor. Look straight ahead, opening the front of your chest.

6 Now it's time for Full Locust. On your next inhalation, lift up your arms, upper body, and legs, being sure you don't push yourself too high. Instead, come up to a comfortable point and continue to breathe deeply, raising and lowering your body with each breath. Hold for a few breaths and come down on an exhalation.

Modifications, Variations, and Props

▶ There is no beginner modification for this pose. If you find that it strains your back in any way, simply keep your arms and legs closer to the floor.

▶ This pose sequence is traditionally done with your arms underneath your torso, palms against the floor. It's incredibly uncomfortable for most people, but if you want to challenge yourself, you can try it that way. Try to keep your arms as close together as possible under your body, as well as firmly against the mat as you raise your legs. It's tough!

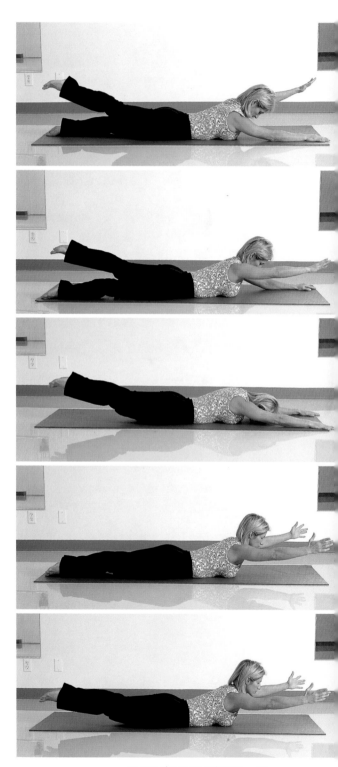

TO SEE THINGS DIFFERENTLY

Dolphin/Easy Scorpion

Go upside-down! It's a great mood lifter, and if you can laugh at yourself (and I certainly hope you can) you'll have fun while you challenge yourself in these two postures. One of these poses, Scorpion, is about as tough as yoga gets. (In a true Scorpion pose, you wouldn't rely on a wall for support. Instead, you would swing your legs up over your head. Flexible yogis are actually able to bend their legs and bring their feet to their head.) But don't worry—we'll be doing an easy, supported version. The goal here is to change the way you're looking at yourself, your worries, and the world in general. Turning the world on its head is a physical reminder that everything is not always as it seems.

Moving Through

If you were doing these two poses together in their most challenging versions, you would be moving from a push-up with your forearms down to a headstand, also done from the forearms. But we're not going to do quite that much. In our version, we're simply going to move from a modified push-up position—it looks like a variation of Downward Facing Dog—to a forearm balance that allows you to use one foot to remain steady. Hold each pose for about 10 seconds and go through the whole series a total of 10 times.

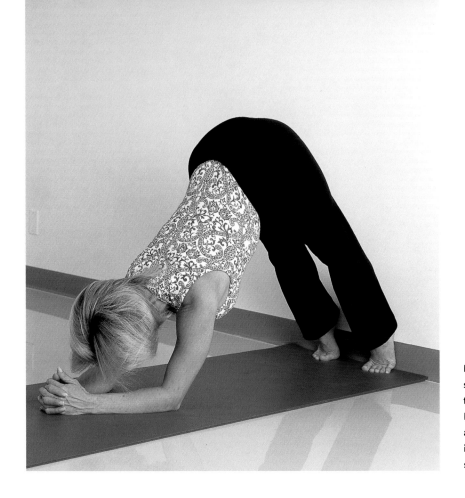

Dolphin stretches the hamstrings, calves, back, gluteus, shoulders, and neck. It also strengthens the forearms, back, and shoulders; improves posture; and stimulates the thyroid.

1 Start with your feet about 1 foot from a wall, hands on the floor directly below your shoulders and knees directly below your hips. Your shins and the tops of your feet rest against the floor. Keep your fingers splayed, but not clenched. Be sure your back is neither arched nor swayed. Your pelvis and neck should be in neutral, eyes looking to the floor.

2 Breathing normally, lower to your forearms. Let your back tilt naturally at an angle, but don't allow it to sway or arch.

3 Push your tailbone back, straighten your legs, and drop your head between your arms, crown toward the floor. Come up on your toes and press the soles of your feet against the bottom of the wall. This is Dolphin; it will look like a modified Downward Facing Dog pose.

continued on the next page >

TO SEE THINGS DIFFERENTLY

Dolphin/Easy Scorpion *(continued)*

4 Hold for 10 seconds.

5 Remain on your forearms with the bottoms of your feet against the wall. Keep your legs straight as you begin to walk your feet up the wall (you may need to move further away from the wall). Keep your back straight, and don't collapse your shoulders.

6 Bring your legs as close to parallel with the floor as you can, staying straight and strong. Hold for 5 to 10 breaths, then walk your legs back down and into Dolphin. Repeat the series 10 times.

Modifications, Variations, and Props

▶ If you have trouble keeping your knees straight in Dolphin, feel free to bend them a little. That should allow you to get your back even straighter. (The pull of both sets of limbs at one time is what makes the pose so difficult.)

▶ If your shoulders are tight and you can't get your forearms comfortably to the floor, use blocks or a folded blanket to elevate them.

▶ If you want something more challenging than the modification above but you can't get into a full Scorpion (and it's a very advanced pose), you could face the wall at the beginning of the pose and, when you swing your legs up, let your feet touch the wall for balance.

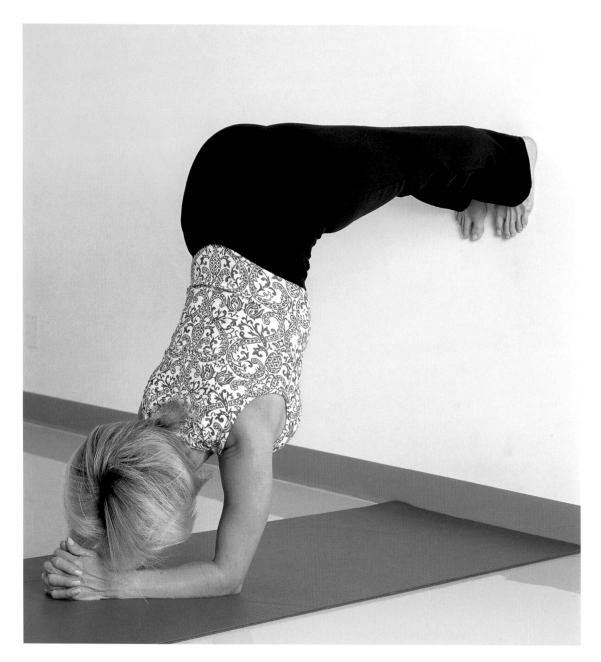

Scorpion strengthens the arms and improves balance, increases blood flow to the brain and pituitary gland, and revitalizes all of the body's systems. It also improves mood while stretching the spine, improving spinal flexibility, and increasing body-mind coordination.

TO IMPROVE YOUR MOOD

Side Prayer Series

This series of poses will put a smile on your face in two ways. First, it asks your body to do a whole bunch of things at one time: stay grounded, twist, reach high with your torso, and acknowledge inner peace by placing your hands in Prayer position. Second, the twisting and turning will force your mind out of the doldrums, allowing it to find a happier, more serene state.

1 Begin in Mountain with your feet hip-width apart. Bring your hands into Prayer position just in front of your heart. Press your hands together firmly, feeling the muscles in your back stretch and your chest compress. Keep your shoulders relaxed. Begin to go into Chair, trying to make your thighs parallel to the floor and leaning forward over your thighs. Be sure to keep your butt tucked under, and don't let your lower back sway.

2 As you move deeper into Chair, begin to twist your torso—without moving your hips—to the right. Bring your right elbow back as far as possible and bring your left elbow to the outside of your right knee. Keep your neck straight. Make sure your feet are grounded and your hips are pulled straight while your torso twists, and that your right side stretches with your right elbow. Your neck should be elongated, with the crown of your head reaching toward the sky. Your eyes can look straight in front of you or up, whichever feels more natural. Hold for 5 breaths.

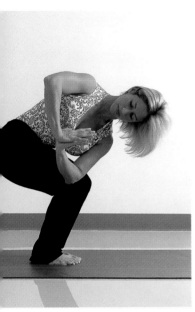 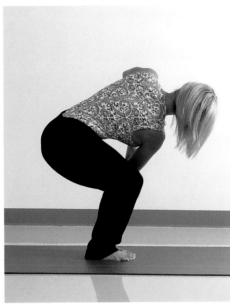 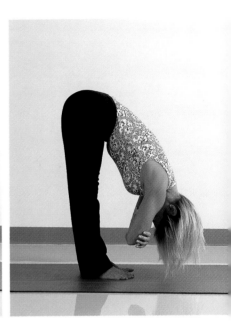

This series stimulates the internal organs; strengthens the quadriceps; and stretches the gluteals, hamstrings, and calves. It also stretches the spine and upper back muscles while strengthening the shoulders and easing tension in the spinal column and neck.

3 Return slowly to the center, and twist to your left side. Use your left elbow to pull your torso to the left, bringing your right elbow to the outside of your left knee. Keep your back straight and your neck long. Keep your feet grounded and hips straight. Hold for 5 breaths.

4 Return to the center position (Chair) and grasp your left elbow in your right hand and vice versa. Drop forward into Forward Bend, being sure to keep your abdominal muscles contracted and your butt pointing to the ceiling. Take a few breaths.

continued on the next page >

TO IMPROVE YOUR MOOD

Side Prayer Series (continued)

5 Now go into Extended Side Prayer. Begin in Mountain with your hands in Prayer. Move into Chair and then into Side Prayer to the right, continuing to breathe deeply. Once you've come into full Side Prayer, reach your right arm up and your left arm down. Your right arm should pull back a bit, but it shouldn't fall back; use its strength to keep it long and upright. Press your left arm against the lower part of your right leg. Use that resistance to keep your torso straight and flat (you shouldn't be falling to the right). The tough thing here is to keep your hips square to the front and both feet grounded. Keep your shoulders relaxed. Look up. Hold for 5 breaths.

6 Return to Chair. Repeat to the left side for 5 breaths.

7 Return to Chair and drop into Forward Bend, interlacing your fingers behind your back and stretching your arms up and over your head. Hold for a few breaths.

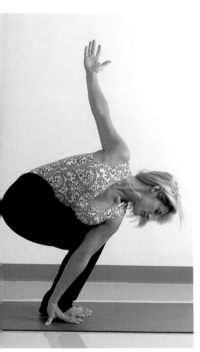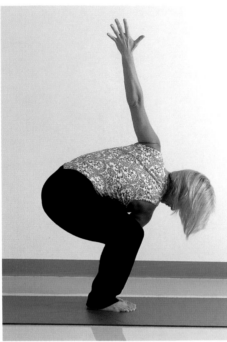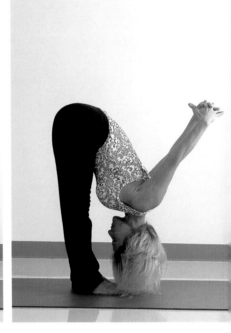

Modifications, Variations, and Props

▶ Although Side Prayer is considered a fairly easy pose, it's quite deceptive. When done correctly, your torso will twist completely over your hips, which should remain stationary and straight. The twisting sensation should be your focus and you should try not to fall or collapse in your back or legs.

▶ If you want to go into Extended Side Prayer but have difficulty reaching your arm far down your leg, place a block beside your foot and lean on that.

▶ Ask a friend to check your form to make sure your torso is straight and not tilted. Each section of your body—your hips/legs and your arms/torso—should be on its own flat plane. There should be no leaning or tilting.

TO NURTURE YOURSELF

Child's Pose

Usually used as a restorative pose to do between other, more-challenging poses, you can do Child's Pose on its own, too. I find it particularly comforting when I've been putting out a lot of energy, such as when I'm taking care of my son or cleaning. This pose allows you to come back into yourself, and it rests your back, legs, and neck in a very gentle manner.

1 Kneel on the floor. Touch your big toes together and sit your butt on your heels with your back straight. Tuck your butt slightly under, so that your back isn't swaying. (Even though this is a relaxing pose, you'll want to start with your muscles engaged.)

2 Exhale and lay your torso down over your thighs, hands stretched out in front of you, palms down. Broaden your sacrum across the back of your pelvis. Lengthen your tailbone away from the back of your pelvis while you lift the base of your skull away from the back of your neck.

3 Either focus on relaxing completely, letting your back melt over the support of your legs, or focus on feeling strong in this pose by keeping your legs together and quadriceps taut, and by imagining lengthening your spine from top to bottom.

4 Lay your hands on the floor alongside your torso, palms up, and release the fronts of your shoulders toward the floor. Grab the outsides of your feet and feel how the weight of your shoulders pulls your shoulder blades wide across your back.

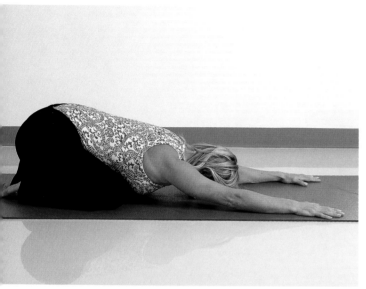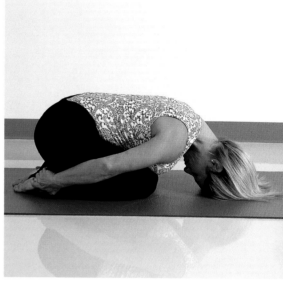

Child's Pose stretches the hips, thighs, back, neck, and ankles. It also relieves stress, headaches, and neck and back pain, and can ease anxiety.

5 Stay in this pose for 30 seconds to a few minutes. To come up, first lengthen your front torso, and then inhale and lift from your tailbone as it presses down and into your pelvis.

Modifications, Variations, and Props

▶ If you have difficulty sitting on your heels in this pose, place a blanket between the backs of your thighs and your calves.

▶ To increase the length of your torso, stretch your arms forward and lift your buttocks just slightly away from your heels. Reach your arms longer while you draw your shoulder blades down your back. Then, without moving your hands, sit your buttocks down on your heels again.

TO FEEL PROUD

Boat

It isn't easy, but I think it's very important, especially when you're feeling sad or scared, to remember that you are still a person who can accomplish things and that you should feel proud of yourself. It actually takes a lot of courage to try to fight your depression and anxiety, so pat yourself on the back. It might take you a while to build up enough abdominal strength to do this exercise—Boat is a toughie, and it really challenges the abs—but once you've gotten it, you'll not only feel strong and beautiful, you'll look strong and beautiful, too! The lines of this pose are truly elegant.

1 Sit on the floor with your legs straight out in front of you. Press your hands on the floor a little behind your hips, fingers pointing toward your feet, and strengthen your arms. Lift through the top of your sternum and lean back slightly. As you do this, make sure you don't round your back; continue to lengthen the front of your torso between your pubis and top sternum. Sit on the "tripod" of your sitting bones and tailbone.

2 Exhale and bend your knees, then lift your feet off the floor, so that your thighs form about a 45-degrees angle with the floor. Lengthen your tailbone into the floor and lift your pubis toward your navel. If possible, slowly straighten your knees and raise the tips of your toes slightly above the level of your eyes as you stretch your arms out alongside your legs, parallel to the floor. If this isn't possible, keep your knees bent and try lifting your shins parallel to the floor, holding the backs of your thighs, if necessary.

3 Spread your shoulder blades across your back and reach strongly out through your fingers. If your hands are grasping the backs of your thighs, hold the muscles in your arms firm.

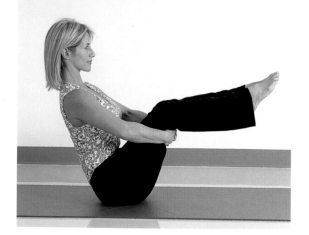

This pose strengthens the abdomen, hip flexors, and spine and stimulates the kidneys, thyroid and prostate glands, and intestines. It also helps relieve stress and improves digestion.

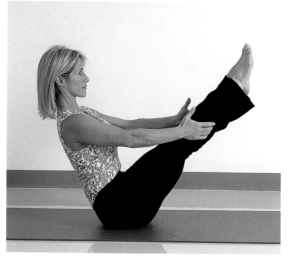

Modifications, Variations, and Props

▶ If it's difficult to straighten your raised legs, you can try this pose with just one leg raised or you can do it without raising up so far off the ground. Gradually work toward performing the unmodified pose as you build up your strength.

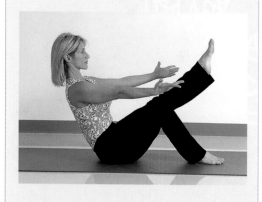

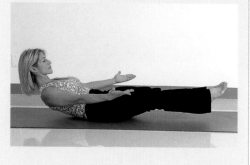

4 Keep your lower belly firm and relatively flat, but not hard and thick. Breathe easily. Tip your chin slightly toward your sternum so the base of your skull lifts away from the back of your neck.

5 Begin by staying in the pose for 10 to 20 seconds. Gradually increase the time until you can hold the pose for 1 minute.

6 Release your legs with an exhalation and sit upright on an inhalation.

TO GET UNSTUCK

Dancer

This is my favorite pose of all, because it looks gorgeous, feels great, and is just difficult enough that you can feel proud of yourself when you're doing it, but not so difficult that you can't learn it quickly.

It's often hard to stop negative thoughts from spiraling out of control when you're sad or nervous, but this pose, with its focus on both sides of the body, forces both sides of the brain to work together, thus taking the focus off your worries.

1 Stand in Mountain with your feet slightly apart and legs strong. Find a point on the floor or on the wall in front of you to focus on. Bend your right knee, bringing your right foot behind you, while you keep the weight of your body on your left leg. Turn your right hand palm out, and place your right foot in your palm. Bring your left arm straight out in front of your body, palm facing forward.

2 Straighten your torso again and be sure your left foot is planted firmly on the floor. Now, with a slow exhalation, begin to lift your right foot and leg up and out toward the back while you also stretch your left arm forward, tilting your torso and head down. Your goal is to stretch in every direction—your left arm is pointing far away from your torso, your right arm is helping your bent leg to stretch as much as possible, and your legs are "splitting" away from each other.

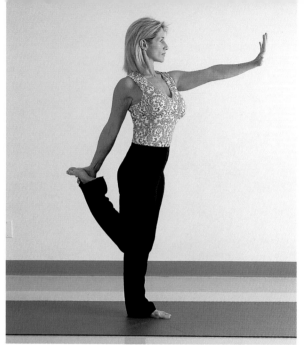
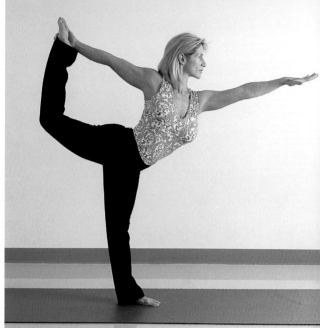

3 Take a few breaths in this position, keeping your eyes focused on the point on the floor.

4 Return to Mountain and repeat to the other side.

This pose improves balance, focus, and concentration. It stretches the hips, legs, back, and shoulders while it strengthens the abdominal muscles.

Modifications, Variations, and Props

▶ This is a pose that intimidates many new yogis; they can't imagine balancing on one leg, and forget about stretching their legs that far apart. The important thing in the pose is to try to remain relaxed while you balance, rather than worrying about how straight you are or how high your leg is. You'll get there, so the first time you do the pose, feel free to keep your standing leg slightly bent, or even do it in front of a wall or chair so you can touch it lightly if you feel yourself falling out of the pose. I believe that it's much better to get used to how the pose should feel rather than worrying about doing it perfectly right away.

▶ Some people like to move quickly into Dancer while others, like me, take their time in each position, finding their balance each step of the way before moving slowly into the full pose. Experiment and see what works for you. Either way, the most important thing is to find your focus before you move and keep that focus throughout the entire posture.

TO BE OKAY EVEN IN A CROWDED ROOM

Half Lotus/Cobbler With Mudra

Although many of us think of depression and anxiety as being a lonely problem—as in "I feel very alone"—the sad truth is that many of us feel sad and anxious in a crowded room. I had one of my worst anxiety attacks in a classroom, and I kept having to leave the room every five minutes to try to calm down. This pose is meant to solve this problem. The key is to use the mudra (hand pose) almost as a hypnosis tool. You'll put your hands into a specific position, such as left hand in right palm, to help physically remind yourself that you are safe and calm. The beauty of this is that no one knows you're doing it. Also, if you can, use the mudra to remind yourself to breathe deeply and, if possible, you can call upon the White Light Meditation (see page 40) to further relax.

Cobbler Pose With Breaths

Bound Angle Pose, also called Cobbler's Pose after the typical sitting position of Indian cobblers, is an excellent groin- and hip-opener.

1 Sit with your legs straight out in front of you, raising your pelvis on a blanket if your hips or groin are tight. Exhale, bend your knees, and pull your heels in toward your pelvis. Drop your knees out to the sides and press the soles of your feet together.

2 Bring your heels as close to your pelvis as you comfortably can. With your first and second finger and thumb, grasp the big toe of each foot. Always keep the outer edges of your feet firmly on the floor. If it isn't possible to hold your toes, clasp each hand around the same-side ankle or shin, or rest your hands in your lap.

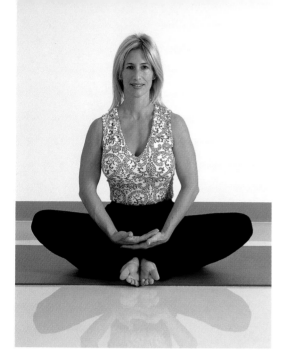

This pose stimulates the abdominal organs, including the ovaries or prostate gland, bladder, and kidneys. It stimulates the heart and improves general circulation while it stretches the inner thighs, groin, and knees. It also helps relieve mild depression, anxiety, and fatigue, and it soothes menstrual discomfort and sciatica.

Modifications, Variations, and Props

▶ To release your thighs, fold two blankets and put one under each outer thigh, supporting your thighs an inch or so above their maximum stretch. Then lay a 10-pound sandbag on each side of your groin, parallel to the crease between your thigh and pelvis. Release your thighs away from the weight, letting them sink into the blankets. Note: Do not use the bags unless your thighs are supported.

▶ Exhale and lean your torso forward between your knees. Remember to come forward from your hip joints, not your waist. Bend your elbows and push them against your inner thighs or calves (but never your knees). If your head doesn't rest comfortably on the floor, support it on a block or the front edge of a chair seat.

▶ If this pose is difficult for you and your knees are very high and your back rounded, sit on a high support—as high as a foot off the floor.

▶ Imagine you have two partners, each pressing inward (toward your pelvis) on a knee. From the middle of your sacrum, push out along your outer thighs against this imaginary resistance. Then push your heels firmly together from your knees.

3 Sit so that your pubis and tailbone are equidistant from the floor. Your perineum will then be approximately parallel to the floor and your pelvis in a neutral position. Firm your sacrum and shoulder blades against your back and lengthen your front torso through the top of your sternum.

4 Never force your knees down. Instead release your thighbones toward the floor. Your knees will follow.

5 Stay in this pose for 1 to 5 minutes. Then inhale, lift your knees away from the floor, and extend your legs back to their original position.

Half Lotus

Full-Lotus brings both feet onto the upper thighs—a tough thing for even the most flexible of yogis! However, Half Lotus allows you to sit in a relaxed, yet challenging position. One that, for many yogis, is highly relaxing. Try not to sit with the same leg on top each time. Try to alternate for more balance in the back and thighs.

1 Sit on the floor with your legs straight out in front of you. Bend your knees and, as you begin to cross your legs, bring your right foot above your left upper thigh.

2 Lean back slightly as you bring your right foot to rest on your left thigh. Be sure to keep both hips resting on the floor, your abdominal muscles contracted, and your shoulders lowered, so there is no tension in your body.

3 Place your hands in the mudra position that feels best for you.

Modifications, Variations, and Props

▶ In Full Lotus, both feet rest on the opposite upper thighs. As you sit this way, be sure to lift your chest and lengthen your back and crown of your head.

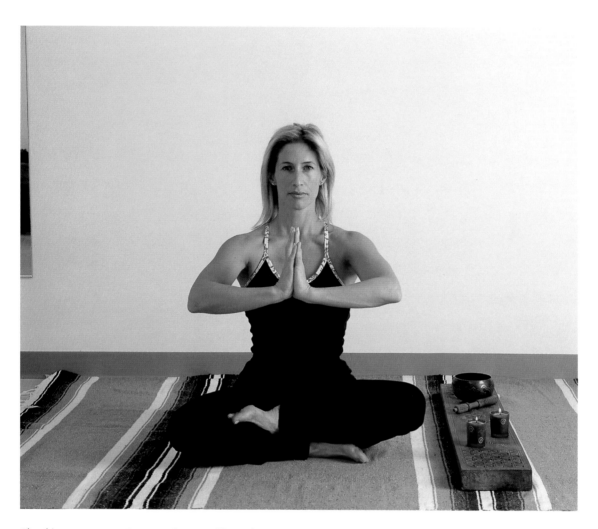

The ultimate yoga pose, Lotus requires open hips and consistent practice to improve posture.

Mudras

A mudra is a hand position with a purpose. If it sounds esoteric, think of the way most of us pray—or at least the way we picture prayer: palms gently touching, resting in front of our heart, with our head bowed. This pose—hands touching in front of heart—is actually a mudra called Namaste (pronounced NAH-ma-stay). This is the Prayer pose of yoga, and it means "I bow to the divine in you as you bow to the divine in me." It is a universal symbol of love and respect, both to the divine and to a person, because it acknowledges that the divine exists in each of us.

Mudras can be seen on statues of the Buddha from thousands of years ago. If you look at images of Buddha, you can see that he often has his index finger touching his thumb or his hands resting gently together. Each of these postures has a specific meaning. When you do them, you should have an intention (such as to create a feeling of relaxation or to show your respect to someone) and you should also be open to the pose's gift. For example, simply putting your hands in Namaste immediately brings me a feeling of serenity. It is a little reminder that the divine is right here, even when I'm busy performing little daily tasks.

Of course, there are other mudras for other intentions. I am particularly fond of touching my thumb tips together and I also love to place my left hand in my right palm. When I do this, even if I am sitting in a co-worker's office or driving in traffic, I am instantly reminded that I have a white light within me and that—even though I cannot go into Lotus or practice Downward Facing Dog—the spiritual and psychological elements of those poses are available to me, right here and right now.

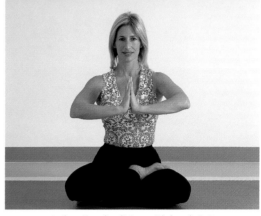

Namaste: A "bow" to the divine, with hands in Prayer pose in front of your heart.

Incidentally, it wasn't a yoga teacher who taught me the power of mudras, it was a psychiatrist. After I was released from the hospital, my doctor was a cognitive psychologist whose job it was to teach me how to think differently, to be hopeful. This doctor was different from all of the therapists I'd seen in the past because she didn't ask me to focus on my past, on my feelings, or even on what I'd just been though. Instead, Betsy had me get through the next day or the next week by visualizing what I wanted to happen. And during my visualizations, she asked me to find a way to hold my hands. I chose to put my left hand in my right, with my thumbs touching. Each time I held my hands this way, my doctor assured me, I would relax, and remember the relaxed feeling I had in her office.

She was right. It worked.

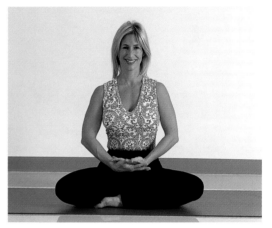

Gesture of Meditation: This posture allows for restful thought and mindfulness. One hand rests gently in the other, and you can touch your thumbs together to encourage a feeling of connection.

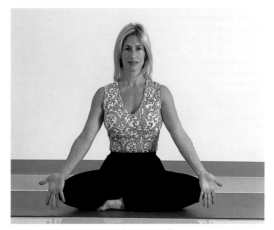

Gesture of Reception: (palms open, fingertips toward the ground) This pose encourages you to open yourself to the goodness around you and to be receptive to the world's gifts. In it your palms are open and your fingertips point toward the earth, grounding you in the here and now.

Namaste

① Sit comfortably in Lotus, your thumbs lightly on your sternum.

② Press your hands firmly but evenly against each other. Make sure that one hand (usually your dominant hand) doesn't overpower the other. If you find such imbalance, release the dominant hand until both hands are pressing equally.

③ Bow your head slightly. Lift your sternum into your thumbs and lengthen down along the back of your armpits, making your back elbows heavy.

Modifications, Variations, and Props

▸ To help widen your sternum and collarbones, press a block or book (3 to 4 inches thick) between your palms. Spread the skin of your palms and stretch your fingers out of the centers of your palms. Then recreate this same width without the block, palms touching.

▸ This palms-together gesture is usually centered over the heart, but you can also raise your pressed hands to the front of your forehead or bring them slightly above and in front of the crown of your head.

Mudras reduce stress and anxiety; calm the brain; create flexibility in the hands, fingers, wrists, and arms; and open the heart.

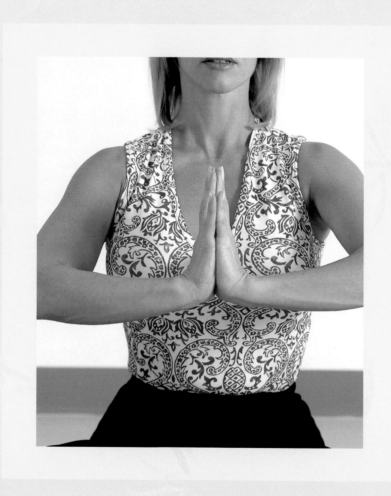

POSE WITH A SMILE

Seated Twist With 10 Breaths

I saved this pose for last, not because it is the most strenuous or the most elegant, but because it is a reminder. I always teach it toward the end of my class, and when I tell my students to smile they always laugh because so few of us think it's okay to smile during yoga or during so much of our lives—at work, in church, wherever.

Smiling, just the act of turning your lips up, has actually been shown to improve mood. And while I'm not suggesting that you should smile through your troubles or ignore any real feelings of the blues, I do believe that remembering to smile, even when faced with a difficult situation, will help you face any problem with hopefulness. And hopefulness can be a key part of making a good decision—one that will bring us greater happiness.

This pose strengthens and stretches the spine and gluteals; massages the organs; stretches the shoulders, back, and chest; and releases tension.

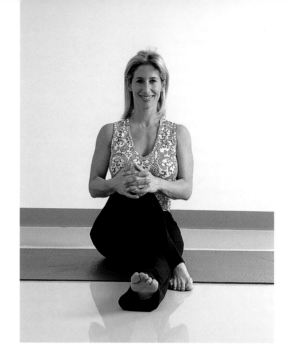

1 Sit on your butt with your legs extended out in front of you, back straight, and shoulders down. Bend your right knee and put your foot on the floor on the outside of your left leg. Keep your left leg strong and rotated slightly inward. Press your thighbone to the floor.

2 Bend your left leg under, but make sure that you are still balanced on both sitting bones. Also press your inner right foot actively into the floor, but soften your inner right groin to receive the pubis as you twist. (Grounding the bent-knee foot will help you lengthen your spine, which is always the first prerequisite of a successful twist.)

3 As you exhale, rotate your torso to your right and wrap your left arm around your right thigh. Hold your outer thigh with your left hand, then pull your thigh up as you release your right hip toward the floor. Press your right fingertips onto the floor just behind your pelvis to lift the torso slightly up and forward.

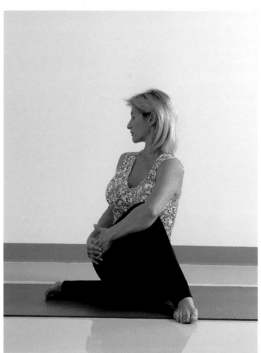

continued on the next page >

POSE WITH A SMILE

Seated Twist With 10 Breaths *(continued)*

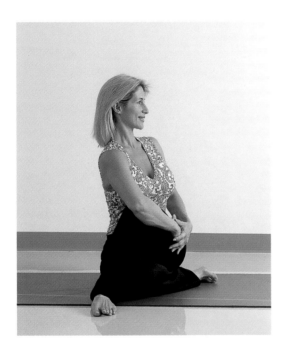

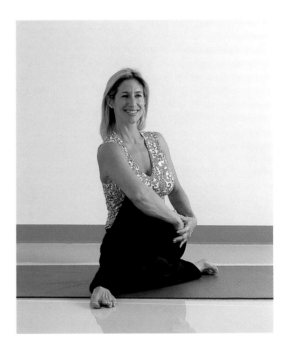

4 Remember to keep your left leg and right foot grounded. Sink your inner right groin deeper into your pelvis, then lengthen your front belly up out of your groin along your inner right thigh. Continue lengthening your spine with each inhalation, and twist a little more with each exhalation. Hug your thigh to your belly, then lean back against your shoulder blades into an upper-back backbend. Gently turn your head to the right to complete the twist in your cervical spine.

5 Stay in the pose for 30 seconds to 1 minute. Then release with an exhalation, reverse your legs, and twist to the left for an equal length of time.

6 Smile.

Modifications, Variations, and Props

▶ Sometimes it's difficult to get your torso in an upright position in this pose, which makes the twist more difficult. Set up the pose with your back about 1 foot away from a wall. After you've twisted, press your free hand against the wall to move your torso up and forward.

▶ In this pose, your head is usually rotated in the same direction as your torso. But it's also possible to rotate your head in the opposite direction from the torso. When you rotate your torso to the right (as described above), try rotating your head to the left and gazing out over your left big toe.

▶ It's often difficult for beginners to sit upright after bending the knee as described in Step 1. Your pelvis tends to sink backward, which rounds your back and could cause back pain. To offset this problem and keep your pelvis in a neutral position, sit on a thickly folded blanket or bolster.

▶ The full version of this pose is appropriate only for experienced students. Perform Step 1. Exhale and twist your torso to the right, and press your right hand on the floor just behind your pelvis. Swing the back of your left shoulder to the outside of your right knee, keeping the left side of your torso snug against the inside of your right thigh. Reach your left arm forward, toward your right foot, and with an exhalation, sweep your arm around your leg and catch your right shin in the crook of your left elbow. Bring the back of your left hand to the outside of your left hip. With another exhalation, complete the twist by swinging your right arm around your back and clasping your right wrist in your left hand. Hold for from 30 seconds to 1 minute, and repeat for an equal length of time on the opposite side.

afterword

I TRULY BELIEVE THAT YOGA BEATS THE BLUES ONLY INSOFAR AS THE PERSON PRACTICING YOGA has the intention to beat the blues. One of my most vivid memories is of the night I was lying in bed at my mom's house just after being hospitalized for depression. I was feeling like a failure because at 32 I was completely and utterly depressed. I had finally accepted that that word—that dreaded word—applied to me.

And then, truly like a light bulb in my head, I had another thought: Well, if I'm depressed now, then I'm going to strive to be happy in the future.

I hate to say this, but I don't think I had ever given a moment's thought to happiness before that moment. I had strived to be successful, to be thin, to have enough money, to get good jobs—all sorts of things—but I had never once thought about being happy.

In fact, as silly as it sounds, I actually had to begin to think about the things that made me happy. Now, I'm not talking about dumb-happy. It's not as if I wanted to spend my life watching *The Three Stooges* and eating cotton candy. I just mean the kind of happy that keeps you feeling warm and satisfied no matter what's going on around you, the kind of happy that protects you from becoming depressed.

Am I saying that the right attitude protects people from depression and anxiety? No, I am not saying that at all. Since I have suffered from depression, I know that it's always possible that I will suffer from it again. Those are the statistics. I am saying that the right attitude may possibly protect people from further illness and, more importantly, even if it doesn't, at least you will have spent your time being happy rather than not!

I am not Forrest Gump—I am a whiner and a complainer. I can get as bent out of shape about traffic jams and spilling coffee as I do about war and abused children. Believe me, I don't always remember to breathe deeply or have time to practice my Sun Salutations when I get up in the morning. However today, as I write this book, I live in a beautiful home and have a fabulous job. My son and I are thriving and I feel better than I felt even before life rocked my boat with wave upon wave of challenge. I still don't have many of the things that I wished for when I was depressed—the things I was sure would bring me happiness. I'm not married, I'm not rich, and, frankly, I could still stand to lose a few pounds. But I am happy. And when I do feel sad, I practice my yoga and my meditation and my deep breathing in an effort to soothe myself and not lose myself down that spiral again.

Depressed people often think it is selfish and somewhat short-sighted to feel happy in what is often a sad (albeit beautiful) world. There are realities to life— death, illness, broken hearts, true tragedy—that sometimes make happiness seem illusory and almost a form of denial.

But I don't believe that. I believe that happiness exists as much as sadness does and that it is only through happiness that we can truly change the world. It is my belief that happiness begets more happiness. Anger toward the world's wrong-doing will not bring freedom to the oppressed, it will only contribute to the aggravation already plaguing humanity.

If you are blue, if you are facing challenges, if you feel hopeless or if you feel sad, I want to reassure you that happiness is possible and that it is your right. If something is blocking your way to feeling happy, then I encourage you to work through and past it in order to feel good so that not only you, but all of us, will be happier, too.

"If in our daily life we can smile, if we can be peaceful and happy, not only we, but everyone will profit from it. This is the most basic kind of peace work."

—THICH NHAT HANH

acknowledgments

I would like to offer my sincere thanks and appreciation to Holly Schmidt and Ken Fund for the opportunity to write this book. Thank you, too, to Janelle Randazza, Brigid Carroll, Silke Braun, and Claire MacMaster for their support and talent through the editorial process. Finally, thanks to Mary Hart for opening her studio to us and for being such a helpful and knowledgeable model.

I want to thank my parents, Bev and Dan Pagano, and Art Raskin for everything they've done for me and for our families.

I would also like to thank my friends Madonna Behen, Kathy Bruin, Victoria Clayton, Susan Dazzo, Dana Longstreet, and Kate Sullivan. I've never been alone in this world since meeting them. They are each warm, funny, and supportive, and they bring a lot of joy into my life.

Thank you, too, to Jim and Linda Kluge and Chris and Laurel Wheeler for their friendship and parenting help.

Finally, I would like to acknowledge my son, James Kaufman. Talk about happiness! He's a bundle of it and I'm the luckiest mom in the world.

about the author

Donna Raskin is a health and fitness writer, as well as a certified yoga teacher and personal trainer. She has been practicing yoga for over 25 years and has taught yoga in California, Pennsylvania, New Jersey, and Massachusetts. She is the co-author of numerous health and fitness books and has contributed to many magazines, including *Shape, Self,* and *Yoga Journal.* Born in Brooklyn, New York, she currently resides in Rockport, Massachusetts.

about the model

Mary G. Hart is the Director of The Iron Crow Yoga Studio and Yoga Teacher Training Program located in South Hamilton, MA. She is a Nationally Certified Muscular Therapist with over 20 years of training in Holistic Health and Wellness, Nutrition, and Yoga Therapeutics. www.ironcrowyoga.com